Clinical Primer of
PSYCHOPHARMACOLOGY

NOTICE

Second Edition

Clinical Primer of
PSYCHOPHARMACOLOGY
A Practical Guide

DONALD M. PIRODSKY, M.D.
Clinical Associate Professor
Department of Psychiatry
State University of New York Health Science Center
Syracuse, New York

JERRY S. COHN, M.D.
Clinical Assistant Professor of Psychiatry
Medical College of Wisconsin
Staff Psychiatrist
Milwaukee County Mental Health Complex
Milwaukee, Wisconsin

McGRAW-HILL, INC.
Health Professions Division

New York   St. Louis   San Francisco   Auckland
Bogotá   Caracas   Lisbon   London   Madrid   Mexico
Milan   Montreal   New Delhi   Paris   San Juan
Singapore   Sydney   Tokyo   Toronto

CLINICAL PRIMER OF PSYCHOPHARMACOLOGY

Copyright © 1992 by McGraw-Hill, Inc.

All rights reserved. Printed in the United States of America. Except as permitted under the United States Copyright Act of 1976, no part of this publication may be reproduced or distributed in any form or by any means, or stored in a data base or retrieval system, without the prior written permission of the publisher.

1 2 3 4 5 6 7 8 9 0 DOC DOC 9 8 7 6 5 4 3 2

ISBN 0-07-105388-3

This book was set in Optima by Beljan, Ltd.
The editors were J. Dereck Jeffers and Lester A. Sheinis;
the production supervisor was Richard C. Ruzycka;
the cover designer was Marsha Cohen/Parallelogram;
the chemical illustrations were provided by Molecular Designs, Ltd., San Leandro, California.
R. R. Donnelley & Sons Company was printer and binder.

Library of Congress Cataloging-in-Publication Data

Pirodsky, Donald M.
    Clinical primer of psychopharmacology / Donald M. Pirodsky, Jerry S. Cohn. — 2d ed.
        p.   cm.
    Rev. ed. of: Primer of clinical psychopharmacology. 1981.
    Includes bibliographical references and index.
    ISBN 0-07-105388-3
    1. Psychotropic drugs — Handbooks, manuals, etc.
2. Psychopharmacology — Handbooks, manuals, etc. I. Cohn, Jerry S.
II. Pirodsky, Donald M. Primer of clinical psychopharmacology.
III. Title.
        [DNLM: 1. Psychotropic Drugs. QV 77 P671c]
    RM315.P53   1991
    615'.788—dc20
    DNLM/DLC
    for Library of Congress   91-2882
                                                                              CIP

To
**Max, Doris, Laura, and Jason
Joe, Bobby, Jennifer, and Hanna**

· · · · · · · · ·

Our Heritage and Our Future

Contents

Preface

This book is an outgrowth of an introductory course on clinical psychopharmacology that I have been teaching to psychiatry residents at the State University of New York Health Science Center at Syracuse for the past 14 years. It is intended to serve as an introduction to the field for beginning psychiatrists and should also prove useful for board review. Psychiatrists not currently familiar with the rapidly expanding field of clinical psychopharmacology may likewise find this text useful.

However, this book was also written with other disciplines in mind. Over the years I have been asked, on numerous occasions, to lecture on clinical psychopharmacology to medical students, residents of specialties other than psychiatry, family physicians, internists, nurses, and clinical psychologists. I realized that there was a need for a concise yet comprehensive, practical, and easy-to-read introductory text to meet the requirements of various health professionals. It is my hope that they will find all or parts of this book valuable.

The book has been organized according to the four major classes of psychotropic drugs, each class comprising one chapter. The chapters, with minor exceptions, have been subdivided into the same categories to provide easy reference. The important pharmacologic and clinical characteristics of the drugs are described for each drug individually. Clear-cut indications for treatment and guidelines for clinical use are provided for each class of drugs. Current diagnostic terminology from the *Diagnostic and Statistical Manual of Mental Disorders*, 3d edition, revised (DSM-III-R), has been used where applicable. Separate sections on side effects and drug interactions have been expanded in the second edition. The use of psychotropic drugs in the elderly and in pregnancy and lactation is also addressed.

I have been assisted in the preparation of this second edition by Jerry S. Cohn, M.D. Dr. Cohn's knowledge and clinical expertise have been invaluable in the updating of this manuscript.

The references provided in the bibliography are primarily other books in the field of psychopharmacology. These books range from brief overviews to comprehensive reviews of the field and in turn provide more detailed references. All are recommended as further reading.

PREFACE

The field of clinical psychopharmacology continues to grow at a rapid pace and is relevant to a wide spectrum of health professionals. Needless to say, several new psychotropic drugs have been introduced since the first edition of this book was published, and these new drugs have been included in the respective chapters. Every effort has been made to keep the text up-to-date, including sections on drugs with new applications to psychiatry. It is our hope that this book will prove to be a useful introduction to this exciting field for physicians and other health professionals.

Donald M. Pirodsky, M.D.
Fayetteville, New York

Acknowledgments

We wish to thank those who directly and indirectly aided in the preparation of this book.

Our teachers and mentors instilled in us the need to continue our academic pursuits long after our formal training ended.

The residents and medical students at the SUNY Health Science Center warmly received the first edition of this book and encouraged the writing of the second edition.

Our patients, perhaps the best teachers, provided us with the inspiration to share our knowledge to help others.

Ms. Shari Carter deserves special thanks. She typed the manuscript from its very beginning to the final draft and did a superlative job. She also provided much-needed moral support and encouragement along the way.

We also wish to thank Ms. Yvonne Clifton, who assisted in the preparation of the diagrams in the text as well as the proofreading.

Lastly, we would like to express our gratitude to the staff of McGraw-Hill for its courteous and professional assistance with the preparation of this book.

Introduction

The modern era of psychopharmacology began with the introduction of chlorpromazine in 1952. Since then, numerous other medications have been developed to treat psychiatric disorders. Many conditions for which there was no satisfactory treatment can now be safely and effectively treated. In the 40 years since chlorpromazine was introduced, psychopharmacologic agents have become the most frequently prescribed group of drugs in the world. It is estimated that between 10% and 20% of Americans use a prescription psychotherapeutic drug during the course of a year. Estimates for the cost of psychotropic drugs have ranged up to $1 billion per year, and these figures continue to increase. Approximately 70% of all psychotropic drugs are prescribed by nonpsychiatrists. Thus, the use of these drugs is a topic of importance for all physicians.

Paralleling the rapid advances in psychopharmacology has been an increase in the body of knowledge in the field of biological psychiatry. New information about the roles of neurotransmitters in psychiatric disorders and the effects of drugs upon them has altered our thinking about the way we treat these disorders and has provided a stimulus for further research. Important progress has been made in better understanding the mechanism of action of psychotropic drugs, which in turn has led to a better understanding of the psychiatric conditions for which they are used.

This book will review the various classes of psychotropic drugs, with an emphasis on clinical psychopharmacology. Pertinent data on the pharmacologic properties of these drugs, including their mechanism of action and pharmacokinetics, will also be presented.

CHAPTER 1

Antipsychotic Drugs

Antipsychotic drugs have also been called major tranquilizers and neuroleptics. The term *major tranquilizer* leads to some confusion, indicating that these drugs might have actions similar to those of the sedative-hypnotic or *minor tranquilizer* class of drugs. In fact, minor tranquilizers such as diazepam (Valium) and the barbiturates have actions qualitatively different from those of the antipsychotic drugs. The term *neuroleptic* can also be somewhat confusing, although commonly used in Europe. Thus it seems more appropriate to classify these drugs as *antipsychotics*, a term that more accurately describes their action and principal use.

One of the earliest antipsychotic drugs used was the Rauwolfia serpentina derivative reserpine. Although it was reported to be effective, problems arose with its side effects of depression and hypotension. The phenothiazine drug chlorpromazine was developed at about the same time and proved to be more effective than reserpine, soon becoming the drug of choice in clinical practice. Since the introduction of chlorpromazine into psychiatry, many other phenothiazines and several other classes of antipsychotic drugs have been developed. All have been attempts to produce a more efficacious drug with fewer side effects. Unfortunately, the ideal drug, one consistently effective in treating psychoses and consistently devoid of side effects, has yet to be developed. However, a promising new antipsychotic drug, clozapine, appears not to produce tardive dyskinesia, the most troublesome side effect of this class of drugs.

At the present time, three separate classes of phenothiazines and six other classes of antipsychotic drugs are available for use in this country. Other antipsychotic drugs are currently used in Europe and Canada but have not yet been approved for use here. Only drugs presently in use in the United States will be discussed in this and all subsequent chapters.

CHEMICAL AND PHARMACOLOGIC PROPERTIES

With the exception of clozapine, all known antipsychotic drugs block post-synaptic dopamine receptors in the central nervous system (CNS). This is their presumed mechanism of action, given our current state of knowledge. The

1

blockade of dopamine receptors in the limbic system is thought to produce the desired antipsychotic effect. However, as none of the presently available drugs is specific for the limbic system, dopamine receptor blockade in other areas of the CNS produces unwanted side effects. Blockade of dopamine receptors in the basal ganglia produces extrapyramidal reactions, whereas the blockade of another dopaminergic tract, the tuberoinfundibular system, causes increased prolactin release by the pituitary. Thus, drugs with antipsychotic activity also have the capacity to evoke extrapyramidal syndromes and increase serum prolactin. It also appears that the ability of antipsychotic drugs to block dopamine receptors is directly correlated with their clinical potency. It is interesting to note that the early antipsychotic drug reserpine did not block postsynaptic dopamine receptors but acted by depleting intraneuronal dopamine.

Although our knowledge of the pharmacokinetics and metabolism of antipsychotic drugs has been best evaluated in the older agents, some generalizations can be made. The absorption of many antipsychotic drugs is erratic, but peak plasma levels are reached about 2 to 4 hours after an oral dose. The liquid or concentrate form of the medications is better absorbed than the pill form. Intramuscular (IM) injection of antipsychotic drugs results in more complete absorption and produces plasma levels about four times that of equivalent oral doses. Thus, 50 mg of chlorpromazine IM would be approximately equivalent to 200 mg administered orally. These drugs are highly protein-bound (most being more than 90% bound to plasma albumin) and highly lipid-soluble. The plasma elimination half-life of these drugs is variable (from drug to drug and in individual patients), but is typically reported as between 10 and 40 hours. Because of this relatively long half-life, antipsychotics need be given only once or twice a day. These drugs are metabolized by microsomal oxidation and conjugation mechanisms in the liver. Chlorpromazine, the most extensively studied, has been postulated to have over 100 metabolites, some of which are active. Haloperidol, on the other hand, has no active metabolites.

Antipsychotic drugs are not addictive and have a low potential for abuse and dependence. Although tolerance often develops to the side effects of these drugs, tolerance to their antipsychotic effect is not prominent. As antipsychotic drugs also have a high therapeutic index (the ratio of a lethal dose to a dose that produces noticeable clinical effects), it is almost impossible for a patient to commit suicide with an overdose of one of these drugs. Even after large overdoses, coma or respiratory depression is rare.

Differences in the chemical and pharmacologic properties of the antipsychotic agents result in clinical differences that often affect our choice of a drug. These differences, as they pertain to the various classes of antipsychotic agents, are discussed in the following sections.

Phenothiazines

The phenothiazine nucleus is a tricyclic structure, the middle ring containing a sulfur atom and a nitrogen atom. Three chemical subgroups are based on differences in the side chain on the nitrogen atom (R_2 position in diagram). These three subgroups are the aliphatics, the piperidines, and the piperazines. In addition to the different side chains, other changes to the basic phenothiazine nucleus occur at the R_1 position. An electron-withdrawing substituent

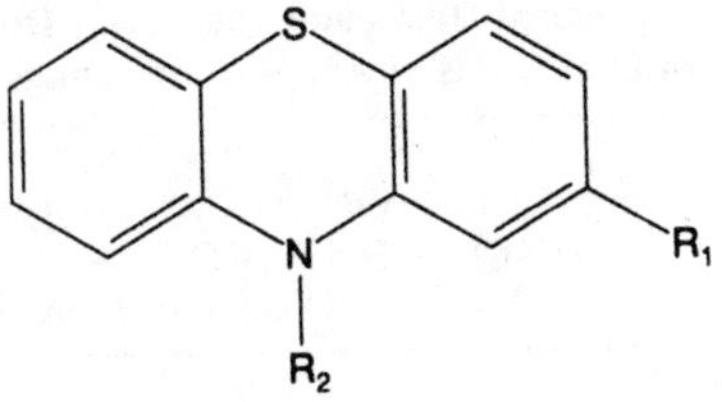

Phenothiazine nucleus

(e.g., Cl, CF_3) must be present in this position for the compound to have significant antipsychotic effects. Certain properties are shared by each subgroup, but important individual differences also exist among the drugs within each group.

Phenothiazines with an aliphatic side chain (e.g., chlorpromazine, triflupromazine) are strongly sedating and also have significant antiemetic and anticholinergic effects. They are potent α-adrenergic blockers and therefore can produce profound postural hypotension clinically. Drugs in this group can produce extrapyramidal syndromes (parkinsonism, akathisia), but do so much less frequently than the piperazine phenothiazines.

Phenothiazines with a piperidine side chain (e.g., thioridazine, mesoridazine) also have significant sedative, anticholinergic, and α-adrenergic blocking effects. Thioridazine is unique in that it has no antiemetic effect. Like the aliphatic phenothiazines, the incidence of extrapyramidal side effects is low with the piperidines.

Phenothiazines with a piperazine side chain (e.g., trifluoperazine, prochlorperazine, fluphenazine) have the strongest antiemetic effects and are the most potent group on a milligram-per-milligram basis (Table 1.1). Sedation, anticholinergic effects, and postural hypotension secondary to α-adrenergic blockade are significantly less with this subgroup. However, they are the worst offenders of the phenothiazines in terms of producing extrapyramidal side effects. In addition to parkinsonism and akathisia, they may also produce acute dystonic reactions, as described in the section on side effects.

Aliphatic Phenothiazines

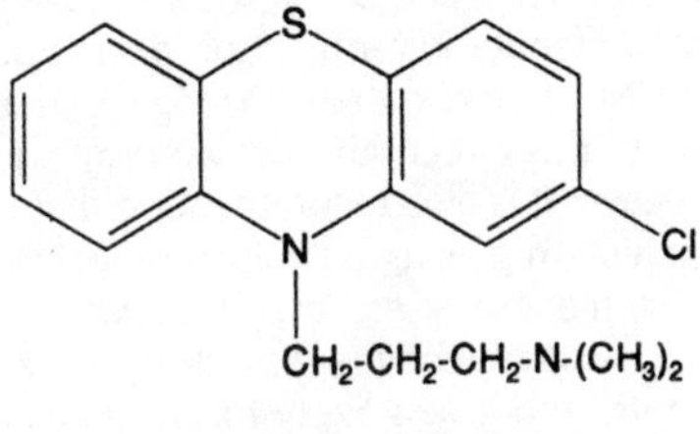

Chlorpromazine

Table 1.1. Equivalent Doses and Usual Daily Dose Ranges of Oral Forms of Antipsychotic Drugs

GENERIC NAME	TRADE NAME	APPROXIMATE EQUIVALENT DOSE (mg)	USUAL DAILY DOSE RANGE (mg/d)	
			ACUTE	MAINTENANCE
Phenothiazines				
Aliphatic				
Chlorpromazine*,†	Thorazine	100	300–1200	100–400
Triflupromazine†	Vesprin	25	75–200	25–100
Piperidine				
Mesoridazine†	Serentil	50	150–400	50–200
Thioridazine*	Mellaril	100	300–800	100–400
Piperazine				
Acetophenazine	Tindal	20	60–160	20–80
Fluphenazine*,†	Prolixin, Permitil	2	6–40	2–8
Perphenazine†	Trilafon	10	16–64	8–24
Trifluoperazine*,†	Stelazine	5	15–60	5–15
Thioxanthenes				
Chlorprothixene†	Taractan	100	300–600	75–400
Thiothixene*,†	Navane	4	15–60	6–20
Butyrophenone				
Haloperidol*,†	Haldol	2	6–100	2–8
Dihydroindolone				
Molindone	Moban	10	40–225	15–60
Dibenzoxazepine				
Loxapine†	Loxitane	15	50–250	20–75
Diphenylbutylpiperidine				
Pimozide	Orap	1–2	2–20	1–10
Dibenzodiazepine				
Clozapine	Clozaril	60	300–900	100–300

*Also available generically.
†Available in injectable (parenteral) form.

Chlorpromazine (Thorazine) is one of the most sedating antipsychotic drugs and probably the worst offender in terms of producing postural hypotension, especially when given IM. No more than 100 mg IM should ever be given at any one time because of this effect, and this amount should only be used if lower doses are ineffective. It is also recommended that no more than 50 mg IM be given at each injection site, as IM chlorpromazine tends to be very irritating and can cause sterile abscesses. After thioridazine, chlorpromazine and triflupromazine are the most anticholinergic antipsychotic drugs. Chlorpromazine is a good antiemetic and is less likely to produce an acute dystonic reaction than prochlorperazine (Compazine).

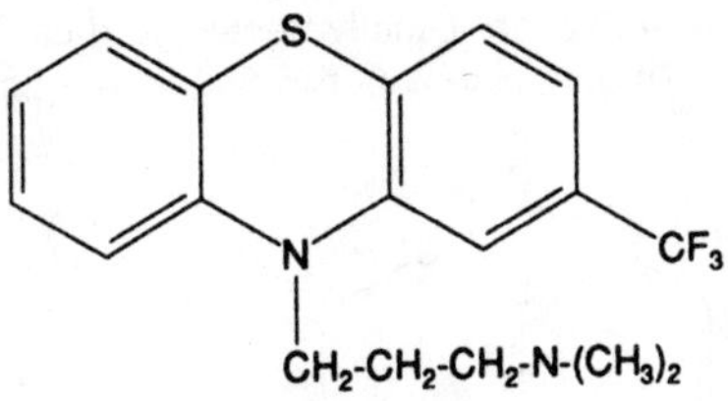

Triflupromazine

Triflupromazine is similar to chlorpromazine, but about four times as potent milligram per milligram. The injectable form comes in 20 mg/mL doses, as compared with 25 mg/mL for chlorpromazine. Thus, fewer milliliters of triflupromazine need to be given to produce an equivalent dose. It is also less irritating than chlorpromazine when given IM.

Piperidine Phenothiazines

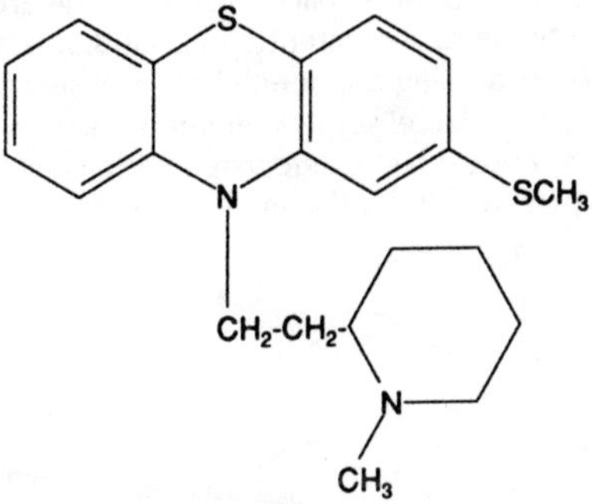

Thioridazine

Thioridazine is the most anticholinergic of all antipsychotics and therefore the one least likely to produce any extrapyramidal side effects. It is the only phenothiazine that does not have an antiemetic effect. It is about as sedating as chlorpromazine and can cause postural hypotension secondary to peripheral α-adrenergic blockade. Because of its potent α-adrenergic blocking effects, thioridazine can inhibit ejaculation or produce retrograde ejaculation, which it does more frequently than any other antipsychotic agent. Because of the risk of pigmentary retinopathy at greater doses, a dose ceiling of 800 mg/d has been established. It is the only antipsychotic drug with an absolute upper-limit dose. Thioridazine is the antipsychotic drug most often associated with electrocardiogram (ECG) abnormalities. The most common ECG changes seen are prolongation of the QT interval, lowering of the ST segment, and flattening and inversion of the T-wave. The appearance of U waves may also be noted, as may prolongation of PR interval. The T-wave changes resemble those seen in hypokalemia, are usually benign, and can be reversed by giving potassium salts. Thioridazine is not available in a parenteral (injectable) form.

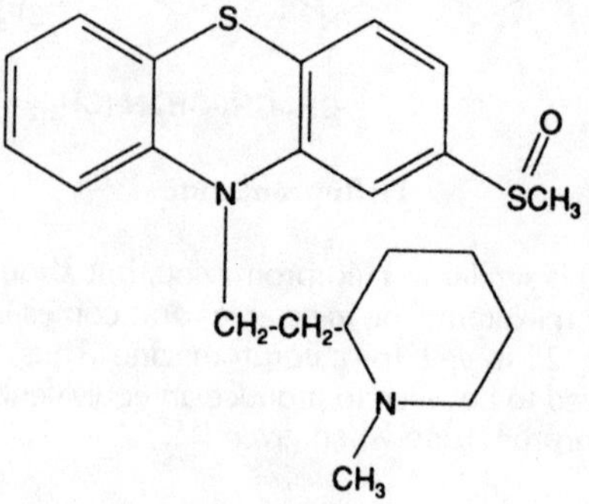

Mesoridazine

Mesoridazine is actually a metabolite of thioridazine and has strong sedative side effects like those of the parent compound. It is about twice as potent as thioridazine on a milligram-per-milligram basis and is available in a parenteral form. It does have some antiemetic activity, and pigmentary retinopathy does not appear to be associated with its use. ECG changes are also less common than with thioridazine.

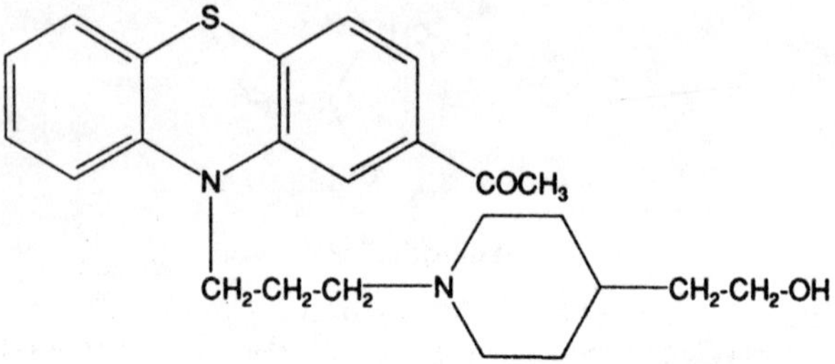

Piperacetazine

Piperacetazine is technically a piperidine, but its structure actually resembles that of the piperazines, and its actions are more similar to that group's. This drug was formerly marketed under the trade name of Quide, but the manufacturer discontinued its production a few years ago. It is no longer available for clinical use.

Piperazine Phenothiazines
This subgroup has the most representative drugs (see Table 1.1). The general comments previously given about this group pertain to all its members. A few of these agents with unique characteristics are discussed here.

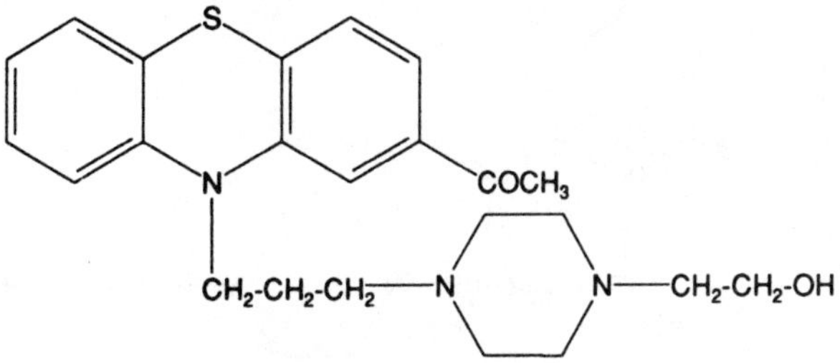

Acetophenazine

Acetophenazine produces the fewest extrapyramidal side effects of any piperazine phenothiazine, therefore it is useful in patients who tolerate such symptoms poorly (e.g., the elderly).

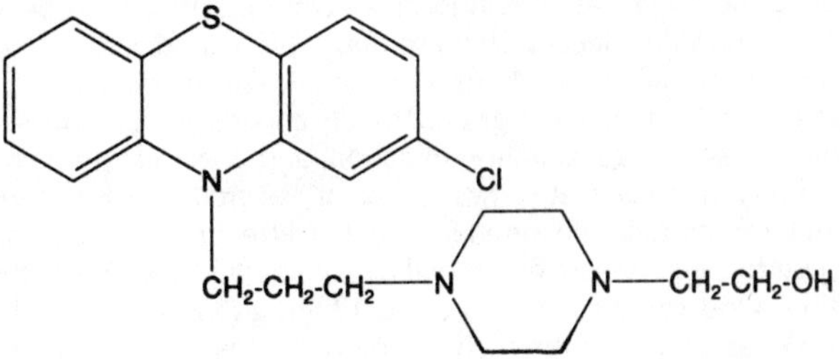

Perphenazine

Perphenazine produces fewer extrapyramidal symptoms (besides acetophenazine) than other piperazines. This is the only antipsychotic agent marketed in combination with a tricyclic antidepressant, amitriptyline. Trade names for the combination are Triavil and Etrafon. Other combinations of antipsychotic and antidepressant drugs are also effective, but the most experience and data are available for this one. Neither agent appears to interfere with the action of the other. Major depressions with psychotic features, in schizophrenic patients, and with severe agitation are indications for this combination. When initiating treatment, the two drugs are generally prescribed separately to give the physician more flexibility in arriving at the right dosage of each. Fixed-combination preparations, such as Triavil and Etrafon, are suitable for maintenance treatment once the dosage has been established. Because of the strong anticholinergic properties of amitriptyline, extrapyramidal side effects are not common with this combination.

Fluphenazine has the highest relative potency of any phenothiazine, being approximately 50 times as potent as chlorpromazine on a milligram-per-milligram basis. It was the first antipsychotic agent in this country to be available in a long-acting injectable form. There are currently two long-acting depot preparations available, fluphenazine enanthate and fluphenazine decanoate. Both contain fluphenazine (25 mg/mL) in a sesame seed oil base. When given

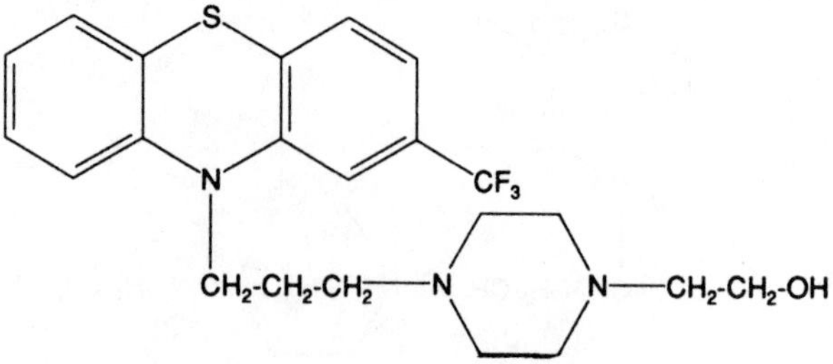

Fluphenazine

IM, the preparation is broken down and the fluphenazine slowly released. The enanthate preparation is effective for 1 to 3 weeks, and the decanoate preparation lasts from 2 to 4 weeks following a single IM injection. These preparations have been invaluable in the treatment of patients who are unreliable about taking their medication and in those who are poor absorbers of oral agents. The main side effects with these depot preparations are extrapyramidal reactions, especially acute dystonic reactions, which generally occur from 1 to 5 days after the injection is given. The decanoate preparation is released more slowly, has a longer duration of action, and generally produces fewer side effects than the enanthate. These preparations are useful for maintenance therapy but are not recommended for the initial treatment of patients. There is no precise formula to convert an oral dosage of fluphenazine to the depot preparation. One study suggested using 12.5 mg (1/2 mL) of fluphenazine decanoate every 3 weeks for each 10 mg daily dose of oral fluphenazine. Other authors recommended giving small test doses (e.g., 1/8–1/4 mL) of these depot preparations and gradually increasing the dosage as tolerated by the patient until the optimal dose is attained. This latter method would seem to provide for better titration of dose to meet each individual patient's needs. Candidates for these preparations should first have a short course of oral fluphenazine treatment to rule out a sensitivity reaction to fluphenazine.

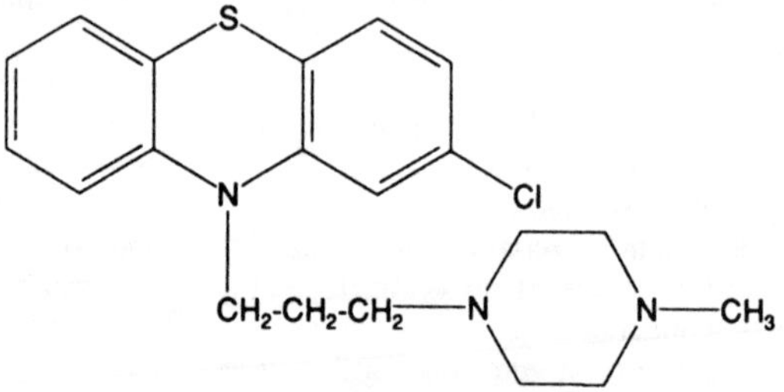

Prochlorperazine

Prochlorperazine, which is marketed under the trade name Compazine, is used to control nausea and vomiting because of its strong antiemetic effects. It is not recommended for use as an antipsychotic agent, since controlled studies have not found it to be as effective as the other phenothiazines. This drug produces mild-to-moderate sedation and is associated with a relatively high incidence of acute dystonic reactions, especially when given intramuscularly.

Butyrophenones

The butyrophenone class of antipsychotic agents is unrelated chemically to the phenothiazines. However, its pharmacologic properties closely resemble those of the piperazine phenothiazines. Butyrophenones are strong antiemetics, have a high relative potency, and cause minimal sedation in nonpsychotic individuals. Their anticholinergic and α-adrenergic blocking effects are also minimal. They have a strong tendency to evoke extrapyramidal reactions, as do the other potent antipsychotic agents.

Haloperidol

Haloperidol (Haldol) is the only butyrophenone approved for use as an antipsychotic in this country. It is an excellent drug for the treatment of acute psychoses and has become widely regarded as the treatment of choice for these conditions. When given IM, it is less irritating locally than chlorpromazine (and other phenothiazines) and also much less likely to produce a serious hypotensive reaction. Also, in contrast to the phenothiazines, haloperidol does not appear to produce any ECG abnormalities. It has been used intravenously in relatively large doses to treat agitated cardiac patients without producing serious side effects. Haloperidol is also available in a long-acting depot preparation, haloperidol decanoate. This preparation is similar to the long-acting fluphenazine preparations previously described. It contains 50 or 100 mg/mL of haloperidol in a sesame seed oil base. The generally recommended maintenance dose is 50 mg IM every 4 weeks, but individual patient needs will vary both in terms of the dose and the time interval between injections. As with the fluphenazine preparations, there is no precise formula to convert oral haloperidol dosage to IM decanoate dosage. A procedure similar to that discussed for the fluphenazine preparations is recommended. Candidates for haloperidol decanoate treatment should first receive a short course of oral haloperidol treatment to rule out a sensitivity reaction to the drug. In addition to its use for treating psychoses, haloperidol is also the drug of choice for the treatment of Gilles de la Tourette syndrome.

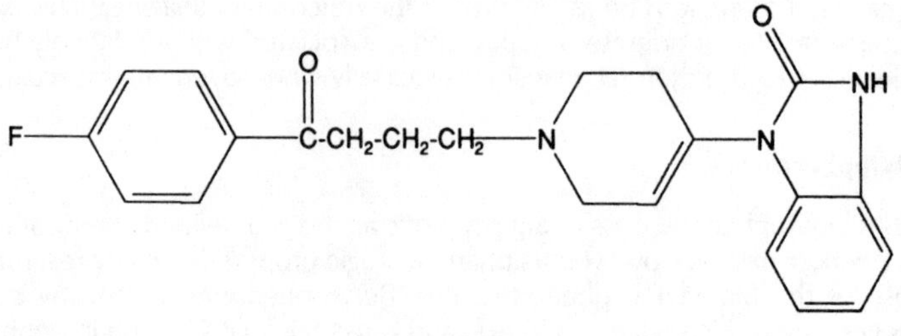

Droperidol

Droperidol, marketed as Inapsine, is used primarily by anesthesiologists for premedication and induction and as an adjunct in the maintenance of anesthesia in this country. It is also used to produce tranquilization and reduce the incidence of nausea and vomiting associated with anesthesia and surgery. It has been reported to be effective in managing excited states from a variety of causes and in Europe is used for its antipsychotic properties. Some clinicians prefer droperidol to haloperidol in the management of acute excited states, as it is more sedating and appears to produce a lower incidence of extrapyramidal side effects. However, it is not approved by the Food and Drug Administration (FDA) for psychiatric use in this country. Droperidol is available only in injectable form in the United States.

Thioxanthenes

The thioxanthenes closely resemble the phenothiazines structurally, the central nitrogen atom in the phenothiazine nucleus being replaced by a carbon atom in the thioxanthene nucleus. As might be expected, their pharmacologic properties are also similar. In general, the modification in the ring of the thioxanthenes tends to make them less potent than the phenothiazines. There are two thioxanthenes currently available for use in this country.

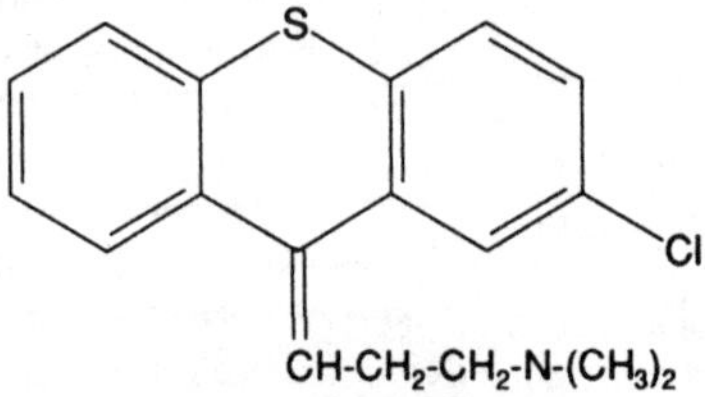

Chlorprothixene

Chlorprothixene is the thioxanthene analog of chlorpromazine and has similar pharmacologic properties. Although it is slightly less potent on a milligram-per-milligram basis than chlorpromazine, it is listed as being equipotent in most tables.

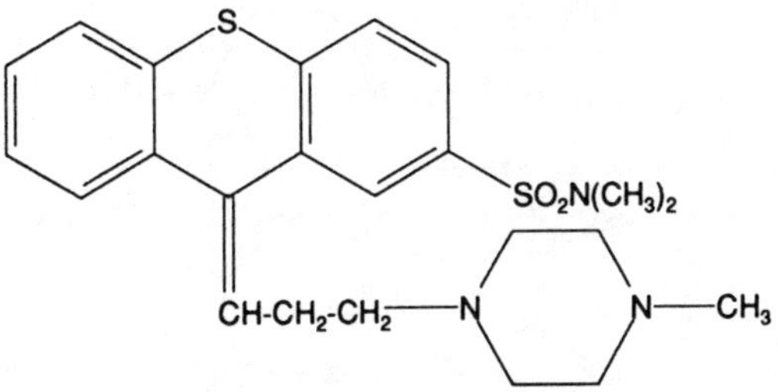

Thiothixene

Thiothixene's chemical structure and pharmacologic actions are similar to those of the piperazine group of phenothiazines. It is one of the least sedating antipsychotic agents. The main side effect associated with its use appears to be akathisia.

Dihydroindolones

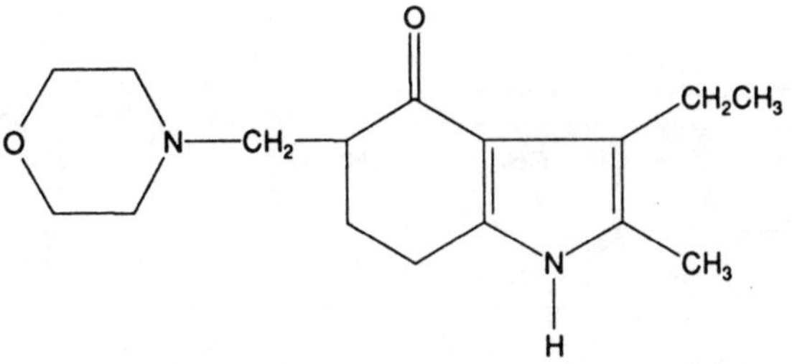

Molindone

Molindone is the only drug of the dihydroindolone class presently in use. It is structurally unrelated to the other classes of antipsychotic agents. It is intermediate in potency and has a relatively favorable side-effect profile. Its sedative effects are intermediate between the aliphatic and the piperazine phenothiazines. Anticholinergic and α-adrenergic blocking effects are mild, as are extrapyramidal side effects. The most common extrapyramidal reaction seen with molindone is an akathisia. Acute dystonic reactions and parkinsonism appear to be less common. Unlike the phenothiazines, which promote weight gain, molindone may actually decrease appetite and facilitate weight loss. Excessive weight gain has not occurred with this drug.

Dibenzoxazepines

Loxapine is the representative antipsychotic of the dibenzoxazepine class. It is chemically distinct from the other classes of antipsychotic drugs. It is intermediate in potency, and its side-effect profile is intermediate between the

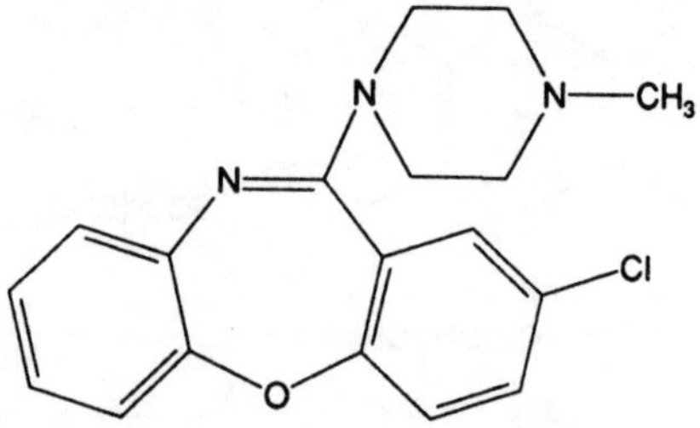

Loxapine

aliphatic and the piperazine phenothiazines. Thus, loxapine may be a useful agent for those patients who have difficulty tolerating the side effects of the high-potency drugs at one end of the spectrum and the low-potency drugs at the other.

Diphenylbutylpiperidine

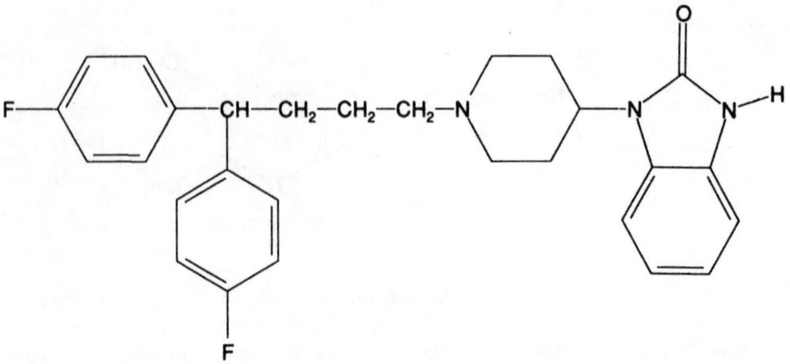

Pimozide

Pimozide, marketed as Orap, is approved for use in this country only for the treatment of Gilles de la Tourette syndrome. However, in Europe it is also used in the treatment of psychoses. Haloperidol remains the treatment of choice for Gilles de la Tourette syndrome, but pimozide may be effective in some haloperidol-refractory patients. It is a very potent dopamine receptor blocker and has a long half-life of 55 hours. Like other potent antipsychotic drugs, pimozide produces unwanted extrapyramidal reactions. Sedation is fairly common, and anticholinergic side effects may occur with its use. However, the main disadvantage of pimozide is its potential to produce cardiac arrhythmias. Like the phenothiazines (especially thioridazine), pimozide produces several ECG changes, including T-wave and U-wave abnormalities and prolongation of the QT interval. Prolonged ventricular repolarization, as noted by a prolonged QT interval on the ECG, increases the risk of developing a potentially fatal ventricular arrhythmia. In cases of sudden death in pimozide-treated patients, this may be the mechanism involved. It is therefore recommended that an electrocardiogram be obtained before initiation of treatment with pimozide and at periodic intervals thereafter, especially during the initial phase of treatment when the dose is being gradually increased. Pimozide should be discontinued if the QT interval of the ECG exceeds 500 milliseconds (470 milliseconds in a child). Because few data are available on the use of pimozide in children under 12 years of age, its use in this age group should probably be avoided. The manufacturer recommends that pimozide be used only in patients with severe symptoms of Gilles de la Tourette disorder who are refractory to or cannot tolerate treatment with haloperidol. Treatment with pimozide should be initiated with 1 mg/d. The dose can then be gradually increased to obtain optimal control of symptoms. Most patients are maintained on doses of less than 0.2 mg/kg/d or on 10 mg/d, whichever is less. The maximum daily dose is 0.3 mg/kg/d or 20 mg/d. Another drug in this class, penfluridol, has the unique property of being effective for almost a week after oral administration. It is not available for use in the United States.

Dibenzodiazepine

Clozapine

Clozapine, which was recently approved for use in this country, is unique among antipsychotic drugs in that it appears to have only minimal antidopaminergic activity. It is referred to by some authors as an "atypical" antipsychotic agent. Clinical trials have shown clozapine to be equal in efficacy (and at times superior) to other antipsychotic drugs. It may be especially useful in the treatment of schizophrenic patients with anxiety, tension, and psychomotor restlessness. The most common side effects seen with clozapine are excessive sedation, orthostatic (postural) hypotension, and hypersalivation. It does not produce extrapyramidal side effects in the recommended dose range (up to 900 mg/d). To date, clozapine has not been associated with the development of tardive dyskinesia, which is its major advantage over the other antipsychotic drugs. Unfortunately, clozapine has been associated with the development of agranulocytosis, and several fatalities have been reported, delaying its approval for use in this country. Clozapine should be considered for use in treatment-refractory schizophrenics or those particularly troubled by extrapyramidal reactions, including tardive dyskinesia. The risk of agranulocytosis warrants weekly blood counts for patients being treated with this drug.

INDICATIONS FOR USE

As the antipsychotics are potent drugs, their use should be reserved for major psychiatric disorders. They are also useful for certain medical and neurological conditions. Their main indications are discussed in the following sections.

Schizophrenia

Schizophrenia is the primary indication for antipsychotic drugs. Schizophrenia is a major psychiatric disorder characterized by delusions, hallucinations, loose associations or incoherence, flat or grossly inappropriate affect, and/or catatonic behavior. Deterioration in work, social functioning, and self-care is prominent. The illness generally begins in adolescence or early adulthood. Some signs of the illness must persist for at least 6 months in order for the diagnosis of schizophrenia to be made.

The antipsychotics are indicated for both acute and chronic schizophrenia. Improvement in both the thought disorder and the degree of agitation or withdrawal is noted in most patients. In other words, these drugs calm agitated schizophrenic patients and activate those who are withdrawn. Improvement in the bizarre behavior of schizophrenics is also noted.

Schizophreniform Disorder

Patients with this disorder display the same features as do those with schizophrenia. However, the duration of this illness is less than 6 months.

Brief Reactive Psychosis

This disorder is characterized by the sudden onset of psychotic symptoms (delusions, hallucinations, incoherence, loose associations, and/or disorganized behavior) following a markedly stressful event. It lasts at least a few hours but no more than 1 month, and there is an eventual full return to the individual's baseline level of functioning. This disorder may not require treatment with antipsychotic medications, especially if the symptoms are mild and of brief duration.

Mania

Antipsychotic drugs are often needed to control acute manic episodes in manic-depressive (bipolar) disorders. Although lithium carbonate is the primary treatment for mania, it has a slow onset of action (approximately 7 days). Thus, an antipsychotic drug may need to be given concurrently until the acute episode is under control. After approximately 7 to 10 days, the antipsychotic drug can be gradually tapered and discontinued, with the patient being maintained on lithium.

Schizoaffective Disorder

Patients with this disorder display features of both schizophrenia and a mood disorder (either a major depressive or a manic syndrome). There is a growing body of evidence that this disorder responds best to a combination of an antipsychotic drug and lithium.

Delusional (Paranoid) Disorder

This disorder is characterized by the presence of a persistent nonbizarre delusion. The delusion is not secondary to an organic factor or any other mental disorder (e.g., schizophrenia). Some patients with this illness respond well to treatment with antipsychotic drugs. Other patients, especially the elderly, may be refractory to treatment.

Organic Mental Syndrome (Delirium and Dementia)

Although the antipsychotic drugs are not the primary treatment for these syndromes, they can be useful adjuncts to the overall medical management of patients with these conditions.

Delirium is an acute confusional state that sometimes follows surgical procedures or placement in a coronary care unit. It may also result from imbalances in electrolytes (e.g., hyponatremia) or other abnormalities of blood chemistry (e.g., increased blood urea nitrogen). The treatment of delirium consists of correcting the underlying cause (where possible), manipulating environmental conditions and at times using antipsychotic drugs to control agitation, excitement, or belligerent behavior associated with confusion and thought disorganization. Sedatives (e.g., barbiturates, benzodiazepines) often aggravate delirium, seemingly by their disinhibiting effects. However, the benzodiazepines are the treatment of choice for the delirium associated with alcohol withdrawal. A delirium or toxic psychosis following the ingestion of a hallucinogenic drug is often self-limiting and requires no pharmacologic intervention. If drug treatment is required, the treatment of choice is generally a benzodiazepine. However, some severe drug-induced psychoses (such as those seen with phencyclidine (PCP)) may require treatment with an antipsychotic drug. When this is the case, treatment with a high-potency agent such as haloperidol is recommended. Many illicit drug preparations contain belladonna alkaloids. The anticholinergic effects of the low-potency drugs (e.g., chlorpromazine) would potentiate those of the belladonna alkaloids and thus compound the toxicity.

Dementias secondary to a variety of causes (e.g., Alzheimer's disease, multiinfarct dementia, trauma) may be accompanied by agitation and belligerent behavior in addition to impairment in memory, judgment, and abstract thinking. If pharmacologic intervention is required to control the behavioral problems associated with dementia, the antipsychotic drugs are often helpful.

Pervasive Developmental Disorders (Autism)

Antipsychotic drugs may be of benefit as an adjunct to psychosocial and/or behavioral therapies in the treatment of autistic children. Symptoms of hyperactivity, withdrawal, aggressive behavior, and stereotyped behavior have been responsive to haloperidol in some studies. However, the response to antipsychotics is often limited, and the clinician must carefully weigh the risks versus the benefits of treatment with these drugs.

Behavioral Problems Associated with Mental Retardation

Antipsychotic medications are often a useful adjunct in the treatment of mentally retarded patients with severe self-injurious behavior, unprovoked assaultive or aggressive behavior, agitation, withdrawal, or uncontrollable hyperactivity. Because of the risk of tardive dyskinesia, the clinical benefit derived from these medications should be well documented and their use should be reviewed on a regular basis.

Major Depression with Psychotic Features

Antipsychotic drugs should not be thought of as having antidepressant effects. In fact, they can make some depressions worse. However, they are an important adjunct to tricyclic antidepressants (or one of the newer agents) in the treatment of major depression with psychotic features. This combination is generally more effective than the antidepressant drug alone. When an antipsychotic drug is used in combination with a tricyclic antidepressant, a high-potency agent (e.g., perphenazine, haloperidol) is recommended. A combination of an antidepressant and an antipsychotic drug is also indicated in the treatment of major depressions in schizophrenic patients and in some severely agitated major depressions. As noted previously, amitriptyline and perphenazine are marketed in a fixed-combination preparation.

Borderline Personality Disorder

Borderline personality disorder is characterized by affective instability, unstable interpersonal relationships, difficulty controlling angry feelings, impulsiveness, instability of self-image, chronic feelings of emptiness, and recurrent suicidal or self-mutilating behavior. There has been increasing evidence that patients with this disorder respond well to low doses of high-potency antipsychotic drugs as an adjunct to psychotherapy.

Gilles de la Tourette Syndrome

This rare disorder, characterized by uncontrolled motor tics, other involuntary movements, barking cries, grunts, and explosive outbursts of obscene language (coprolalia), has been found to respond to antipsychotic drugs, particularly haloperidol and pimozide.

Huntington's Disease

The involuntary choreoathetoid movements of Huntington's disease can be diminished by the antipsychotic drugs, particularly the high-potency agents (e.g., piperazine phenothiazines, haloperidol). However, the antipsychotic drugs do not reverse the progression of dementia or otherwise retard the course of this illness.

Hemiballismus

This extrapyramidal syndrome is characterized by flinging, purposeless movements of the arms. It has been reported to respond to haloperidol.

Nausea and Vomiting

Although prochlorperazine is the most frequently used drug of this class to treat nausea and vomiting, chlorpromazine, haloperidol, and others also have strong antiemetic effects.

Intractable Hiccough

When more conservative measures fail, chlorpromazine has been found to be effective in controlling intractable hiccough.

GUIDELINES FOR CLINICAL USE

Treatment of Schizophrenia

1. Make an accurate diagnosis before initiating treatment with an antipsychotic drug. Be sure that the patient's symptoms are known to be relieved by the medication.

2. The choice of an antipsychotic drug should, if possible, be based on the patient's prior drug-response history. If he or she has responded optimally to a particular drug in the past, that agent should be tried first. Likewise, if a patient did not respond to a certain drug or had an adverse or allergic reaction, that agent should be avoided.

3. If a personal drug history is unavailable, the choice of an antipsychotic should be based on the patient's family drug-response history. Such factors as the absorption, metabolism and receptor sensitivity of a drug can be genetically determined. Thus, if a family member (blood relative) has been effectively treated with a certain drug, the patient should be tried on that agent first. If a family member (blood relative) did not respond to a particular drug or had an adverse reaction to it, that drug should be avoided and the patient treated with another antipsychotic.

4. If neither a personal nor a family drug history is available, the selection of a drug should be based on the side effects that it produces or on its own unique characteristics. For example, substantial sedation may be desirable in an agitated schizophrenic patient but unwanted in one who is withdrawn. Hypotensive side effects would be undesirable in a patient on antihypertensive medication or in the elderly. In a newly admitted, agitated schizophrenic patient who may require large initial doses of an antipsychotic, one would not want to choose thioridazine, which has an upper dose limit of 800 mg/d. For a patient with frequent relapses due to failure to take his or her medication, a trial on a long-acting injectable fluphenazine or haloperidol preparation (e.g., fluphenazine decanoate or haloperidol decanoate) would be appropriate. Molindone could be used in overweight patients, as it may facilitate weight loss. If sedation is undesirable, a high-potency drug such as haloperidol or thiothixene would be preferable. Other examples could also be drawn.

5. Although the antipsychotics vary in potency, they are all effective agents when given in equivalent doses. Thus, potency should not be confused with efficacy. Because so many antipsychotics are presently available, it is unlikely that any clinician would have extensive experience in the use of all of them. It would therefore make good sense for a clinician to pick one or two drugs from each of the three subgroups of phenothiazines and one from each of the other chemical classes and become thoroughly familiar with their clinical effects.

6. Treatment of newly diagnosed schizophrenic patients should be initiated with a single drug. It is often useful to initiate treatment with a small test dose of the drug (e.g., 2 mg of haloperidol orally or 1 mg IM, or the equivalent dose of another drug). This allows the physician to observe the patient for any side effects or allergic reactions. If no adverse effects appear after approximately 2 hours, the dose can then be gradually increased into the effective antipsychotic range (see Table 1.1). The rate at which the dose is increased depends on the clinical condition and overall general health of the patient. As a rough guideline, treatment could be initiated with 300–400 mg/d of chlorpromazine (or an equivalent dose of another drug). The dose could then be increased gradually every 3 to 5 days until an optimal therapeutic response is achieved or troublesome side effects intervene. This treatment is generally done within a 6-week period or less, but patients with exacerbations of chronic schizophrenia may need up to a 3-month treatment period before response should be judged. For young, acutely agitated schizophrenics, the starting dose could be higher and the dosage be increased more rapidly. For older patients or those with concurrent physical problems, lower starting doses and slower rates of increase are indicated.

7. Table 1.1 gives the usual dose ranges for the antipsychotic drugs. Keep in mind that these are average ranges and may not apply to all patients. The individual needs of each patient must be taken into account and the dose be adjusted accordingly. Although some patients may respond to lower doses, studies have consistently shown that doses of chlorpromazine of less than 300 mg to 400 mg/d (or the equivalent doses of other antipsychotics) are ineffective in the treatment of acute schizophrenia. Thus insufficient dosage may be one reason for a failure to respond. Chronic schizophrenics, on the other hand, may be maintained with lower doses.

8. Over the past few years there has been a tendency toward the use of lower doses of antipsychotic drugs. Studies have shown that high doses are no more effective than low to moderate doses and may even be less effective. For example, there are no data to substantiate that doses much above 20 mg/d of haloperidol offer any increased benefit. The technique of "rapid tranquilization," in which patients are given 5 to 10 mg of haloperidol orally or IM every 30 to 60 minutes until their psychosis clears, has recently come under critical review. It now appears that when treatment outcome is measured after a week or more, these patients do no better than patients treated with more standard doses. The occasional patient may indeed benefit from such an aggressive treatment approach, but it is not recommended for routine use. An alternative to high-dose antipsychotic treatment of acutely agitated schizophrenic patients is the use of benzodiazepines in conjunction with moderate doses of antipsychotic drugs. The most commonly used benzodi-

azepine for this purpose has been lorazepam (Ativan) in doses of 1 to 2 mg IM or 5 mg orally. Although controlled studies have not verified the effectiveness of this technique, clinical reports have been encouraging, and it does have the advantage of minimizing exposure to antipsychotic drugs.

9. Initially, it is a good idea to give antipsychotics in divided doses. This tends to minimize the impact of unwanted side effects and allows for better titration of the dose. However, the dose frequency can be reduced once the patient is on a full therapeutic dose regimen. All antipsychotics are long acting and need be given no more than once or twice a day. Ideally, the patient can be given a single daily dose of medication at bedtime. This increases compliance and avoids unwanted side effects. For example, giving one dose at bedtime will aid sleep and avoid excessive daytime sedation. Because plasma levels will peak while the patient is asleep, extrapyramidal symptoms are also less likely to occur. If a divided dose seems more feasible, the majority of the dose can be given in the evening (i.e., give one third of the dose in the morning or afternoon and two thirds in the evening). An exception to this rule is elderly patients, who may not be able to tolerate a single large dose of a drug. They may need a schedule of 3 or 4 doses per day. However, even elderly patients may be able to tolerate small maintenance doses on a once-a-day basis.

10. The first signs of improvement with medication are generally a decrease in aggressiveness, irritability, and restlessness, in addition to an improved sleep pattern. Amelioration of paranoid belligerence and psychomotor retardation are also early signs of improvement. Soon after this point, the patient may become more tractable to treatment and pay more attention to his or her personal hygiene. Later in the course of treatment, hallucinations begin to fade away, and the patient's disordered thinking, perceptual distortions, and social skills all show improvement. Although specific antipsychotic effects may be seen in as soon as 2 days, optimal benefit from antipsychotic drugs may take up to 6 weeks or longer. One of the most difficult aspects to master in the use of antipsychotic drugs is recognizing that improvement generally occurs in phases. In other words, there is a lag period from the time an effective dose is reached until optimal benefit is obtained from the drug. Thus, further increases in dose may not be necessary if the patient appears to be progressing "on schedule." Overall, a satisfactory degree of improvement can be expected in 75% or more of newly admitted schizophrenic patients.

11. Once improvement has occurred and the patient's condition has stabilized (generally in between 4 and 12 weeks), the issue of maintenance treatment arises. The goal of maintenance treatment is to preserve the gains of the initial treatment phase and to prevent a relapse in the patient's condition. An effective maintenance dose is the lowest dose that retains therapeutic gains and allows the patient to function best. To arrive at the maintenance dose, a gradual reduction in the peak dose should be initiated. This reduction should be done over a period of several weeks, as too rapid a decrease may result in a relapse. The eventual maintenance dose may turn out to be roughly one third to one fifth of the peak dose, but there is considerable variation among patients (see Table 1.1). Thus the need to individualize treatment is important.

12. How long to continue maintenance antipsychotic drug treatment is often a difficult question. For the patient with an initial schizophrenic episode,

it has been suggested that maintenance treatment be continued for approximately 6 months. Assuming the patient is in good remission at that time, the drug can be gradually tapered and discontinued. For the patient with a second schizophrenic episode, maintenance treatment for 1 year or more has been recommended. For those patients with three or more schizophrenic episodes, maintenance therapy may be needed indefinitely (or at least intermittently). Studies have shown that maintenance treatment reduces the risk of relapse by about 50%. The clinician must carefully weigh this benefit against the risk of tardive dyskinesia. This issue should be discussed with the patient, and his or her informed consent for continued antipsychotic drug treatment should be obtained. This will be discussed further under "tardive dyskinesia" in the section on side effects.

13. Chronic schizophrenics should be maintained on the lowest possible dose of an antipsychotic drug that will keep their symptoms in remission. Also, periodic (once or twice yearly) attempts should be made to discontinue the drug altogether to see if the patient still needs it. Such a regimen may aid in both the prevention and the early detection of tardive dyskinesia. Many chronic hospitalized schizophrenics maintained on low doses of medication may be getting little benefit from the drugs, which can be safely discontinued.

14. Once it has been decided to discontinue maintenance medication, it is best to gradually taper the dose over a period of several weeks or months rather than to stop it abruptly. This is particularly true for higher maintenance doses. This regimen may allow for early detection of deterioration in the patient's condition before a frank relapse occurs. Should there be any signs of deterioration, the medication could be increased to the last previously effective level.

15. If a newly diagnosed schizophrenic patient does not respond well to maximally tolerated doses of an antipsychotic drug within 6 weeks (3 months for a chronic schizophrenic patient), he or she should be considered refractory to the drug and treated with another antipsychotic. Although these time periods are somewhat arbitrary, they do emphasize the lag period required to obtain optimal therapeutic benefit from antipsychotic drugs. Before deciding that a patient is refractory, make sure that the lack of response is not due to a failure to ingest or absorb the medication. Noncompliance with treatment is often a cause of poor response. Absorption of antipsychotic drugs can be grossly checked by obtaining a plasma level. At the present time there are no established therapeutic ranges for plasma levels of antipsychotic drugs. However, laboratories can provide commonly observed plasma-level ranges, which may be of some value clinically. For example, if a patient is on a relatively high dose of medication and the plasma level is very low, the patient can be presumed to be a poor absorber (assuming compliance is verified). Likewise, a high plasma level in the presence of a poor clinical response would tend to validate that the patient is refractory to the drug. *If an antipsychotic plasma level is drawn, it should be obtained 12 hours after the last oral dose.* Poor absorption may also be checked clinically by giving the patient a short course of IM administration of the drug. If the patient is truly a poor absorber, a trial on a long-acting depot preparation may be indicated. However, oral absorption of another class of antipsychotic drug may be adequate. Failure to respond to treatment should also lead the clinician to reevaluate the patient

diagnostically to make sure he or she is indeed a candidate for antipsychotic drug therapy.

16. If a patient is refractory to any given antipsychotic drug, he or she should be switched to a more potent drug of the same class or to a drug in another class. For example, if a patient is refractory to chlorpromazine, he or she could be tried on fluphenazine, haloperidol, or thiothixene. The patient should not be tried on thioridazine, which is equipotent to chlorpromazine. If a patient has failed to respond to several antipsychotic drugs, the addition of lithium or carbamazepine to an antipsychotic can sometimes enhance the clinical response.

17. Polypharmacy, the use of two or more antipsychotic drugs concurrently, should be avoided. The use of two antipsychotic drugs in combination has never been shown to be more effective than the use of one drug given in appropriate doses. Polypharmacy also increases the risk of drug interactions and side effects, particularly tardive dyskinesia.

18. Currently, there are differing opinions regarding the appropriate use of antiparkinsonian drugs. Some clinicians recommend the prophylactic use of antiparkinsonian drugs during the early stages of treatment to minimize the risk of extrapyramidal side effects, particularly acute dystonic reactions. Other clinicians recommend treating only emergent extrapyramidal side effects. Since antiparkinsonian drugs have their own side effects, a conservative approach to their use would be to treat only extrapyramidal symptoms, should they occur. However, there may be occasions when prophylactic treatment is indicated. If the aggressive use of a high-potency drug is required to control severe psychotic agitation, prophylactic use of an antiparkinsonian medication may benefit the patient. Another indication would be for those patients who are at high risk of developing an acute dystonic reaction following long-acting depot fluphenazine or haloperidol injections. These patients may require an antiparkinsonian drug for 1 week following each injection.

19. In general, antiparkinsonian drugs should be used as little and for as short a period of time as possible. If it is necessary to use antiparkinsonian drugs, they should be discontinued after no longer than 3 or 4 months. Studies have shown that less than 10% of patients will require these drugs after this period of time. Thus, all patients should have a trial period off antiparkinsonian agents to see if their use is still required. Table 1.2 lists the names and dose ranges for the commonly used antiparkinsonian drugs.

20. With the exception of amantadine, antiparkinsonian drugs exert their therapeutic effect by virtue of their anticholinergic activity. Amantadine works as a dopamine agonist. These drugs have shorter half-lives than the antipsychotic drugs and generally should be prescribed on a bid or tid regimen. It is important to keep in mind that the strong anticholinergic properties of these drugs are additive with those of the phenothiazines and other antipsychotic drugs. Thus excessive anticholinergic side effects (e.g., confusion, constipation, urinary retention, and blurry near vision) may occur with their use. This is of particular concern in the elderly, who are extremely sensitive to anticholinergic side effects. In general, it is best to avoid the use of anticholinergic antiparkinsonian drugs in the elderly. Amantadine can be used for those patients in whom the clinician wishes to avoid any added anticholinergic effect. Amantadine might be expected to exacerbate psychotic symptoms or to interfere

Table 1.2. Commonly Used Antiparkinsonian Drugs

GENERIC NAME	TRADE NAME	USUAL DAILY DOSE RANGE (mg/d)
Anticholinergic agents		
Benztropine*,†	Cogentin	1–6
Biperiden*	Akineton	2–6
Diphenhydramine*,†	Benadryl	25–100
Procyclidine	Kemadrin	5–20
Trihexyphenidyl†	Artane	2–15
Dopamine agonist		
Amantadine	Symmetrel	100–300

*Available in parenteral preparation for acute dystonic reactions.
†Available generically.

with the efficacy of the antipsychotic drugs, because of its mode of action. However, this has not generally been a problem clinically. It does appear, though, that tolerance to its antiparkinsonian effects develops over time.

21. The use of supportive psychotherapy, family therapy, occupational therapy, and/or vocational training should not be overlooked in the treatment of schizophrenia. The schizophrenic patient will require much support in readapting to his or her environment.

Treatment of Other Disorders

When used in the treatment of mania, antipsychotic drugs are generally used for only short periods of time, until the patient becomes stabilized on lithium. Acute treatment of mania may require doses similar to those used to treat acute schizophrenic episodes.

Treatment of schizoaffective disorder and paranoid disorder may require a treatment course with antipsychotic drugs similar to that used for schizophrenia. It is important to make sure that the symptoms of these disorders are responsive to the antipsychotic drugs in order to justify their continued use. As in the treatment of schizophrenia, periodic attempts to taper the dose and discontinue the medication should be made.

The treatment of agitation secondary to delirium requires only short-term treatment with antipsychotic drugs until the underlying cause of the delirium is corrected. Use of a high-potency agent such as haloperidol is recommended to avoid the hypotensive, anticholinergic, and sedative side effects that could complicate or exacerbate the delirium. In the treatment of agitation and belligerent behavior secondary to a dementia, treatment with a high-potency drug in low doses is recommended. For example, haloperidol in doses of 1 to 9 mg/d could be used. Because of the irreversible nature of a dementia (as contrasted with that of a delirium), protracted use of medication may be required. Every effort to use the lowest effective dose of the antipsychotic drug should be made. Alternative treatments should also be considered. Some brain-injured patients have responded well to propranolol. Carbamazepine may also be effective in selected cases.

In the treatment of autism, prolonged use of antipsychotic drugs may be indicated. However, because response to antipsychotics is often limited, care must be taken to document the benefits of treatment and the need for continued use of antipsychotic drugs.

The treatment of behavioral problems associated with mental retardation may require doses of antipsychotic drugs similar to those used to treat schizophrenia, depending on the age and physical condition of the patient. The minimal effective dose should be used, and the drugs should be tapered and discontinued periodically to determine if they are still required. Alternative treatments without the inherent risk of tardive dyskinesia should also be explored. For example, lithium, carbamazepine, propranolol, and clonazepam could be equally or more efficacious than the antipsychotic drugs in selected patients. Recent studies have shown propranolol to be effective in controlling the severe self-injurious behavior sometimes seen in patients with autism and mental retardation.

When used as an adjunct to an antidepressant drug in the treatment of major depression with psychotic features, high-potency antipsychotic drugs are generally used in low-to-moderate doses. As the depression resolves, the drugs can be tapered and discontinued along with the antidepressant. However, maintenance treatment may be required for some patients.

Treatment of borderline personality disorder may require long-term use of low doses of high-potency antipsychotic drugs. As with other disorders, every effort should be made to maintain the patient on the lowest effective dose of medication, and periodic attempts to taper and discontinue the drug should be made.

Gilles de la Tourette syndrome often responds well to low doses of haloperidol (e.g., 0.5 to 5 mg/d). Doses higher than 15 mg rarely have to be used. Pimozide can be used for those patients refractory to haloperidol. Clonidine, an antihypertensive drug, has also been shown to be effective in the treatment of Gilles de la Tourette syndrome. As long-term treatment is generally required for this disorder, patients should be maintained on the lowest effective dose of haloperidol or pimozide to minimize the risk of developing tardive dyskinesia. Treatment with clonidine should also be considered, as this drug may be as effective as the antipsychotics with less potential toxicity.

Huntington's disease and hemiballismus may also require protracted treatment with antipsychotic drugs to control effectively the abnormal movements associated with these disorders. Haloperidol has been most commonly used.

The treatment of nausea and vomiting and intractable hiccough will generally be of brief duration, but will often require the use of a parental or suppository preparation of an antipsychotic. Prochlorperazine and chlorpromazine in low doses are most commonly used for these indications. It is important to keep in mind that IM prochlorperazine can cause acute dystonic reactions, as can the suppository form, while IM chlorpromazine can cause pronounced hypotension.

SIDE EFFECTS

Many side effects of the antipsychotic agents have already been mentioned and discussed. A more complete listing with additional comments is presented in this section.

Oversedation

Oversedation is common with the aliphatic and piperidine phenothiazines, chlorprothixene, clozapine, and, to a lesser degree, loxapine. It does diminish over time even without a reduction in dose, as many patients become tolerant to this side effect. It can be minimized by giving the drug in a single dose at bedtime.

Anticholinergic Side Effects

Anticholinergic side effects include dry mouth, constipation, urinary hesitancy, blurred near vision, tachycardia, and erectile disturbances. These symptoms are usually only bothersome and tend to decrease over time as tolerance to them generally develops. However, in rare instances they can be more severe. Urinary retention (especially in older men with enlarged prostates) and infection of a paralyzed bladder may occur. Paralytic ileus, a fulminating oral infection, or an exacerbation of untreated glaucoma can also occur. The aliphatic and piperidine phenothiazines are the worst offenders in terms of producing anticholinergic side effects. As noted previously, most antiparkinsonian drugs also have strong anticholinergic activity.

Orthostatic (Postural) Hypotension

Orthostatic hypotension is produced as a result of α-adrenergic blockade. Aliphatic and piperidine phenothiazines, clozapine, and chlorprothixene most commonly produce postural hypotension. This effect can be particularly problematic in the elderly and may necessitate switching to another drug. Mild cases can often be controlled by instructing the patient to change positions (e.g., from lying to standing) slowly. Severe hypotensive reaction may follow the injection of IM chlorpromazine. If pharmacologic treatment is necessary to reverse this reaction, a pure α-adrenergic stimulator such as metaraminol (Aramine) or norepinephrine (Levophed) is the treatment of choice. Epinephrine, which is both an α- and a β-adrenergic stimulator, should not be used as it could exacerbate the hypotension.

Cardiac Arrhythmias and Sudden Death

Antipsychotic drugs that prolong verticular repolarization enhance the likelihood of developing a potentially lethal ventricular arrhythmia. This is the presumed mechanism for the rare reports of sudden death associated with antipsychotic drugs. Thioridazine and pimozide present the greatest risk for the development of ventricular arrhythmias and sudden death. The ability of these drugs to increase intracardiac conduction time is of particular concern for patients with preexisting cardiac problems and in those who have taken an overdose.

Early-Appearing Extrapyramidal Reactions

Three common early-appearing extrapyramidal syndromes are associated with the use of antipsychotic drugs. These are produced most commonly by the piperazine phenothiazines, haloperidol, thiothixene, molindone, and loxapine.

Acute Dystonic Reactions

Acute dystonic reactions are acute muscle spasms, most commonly involving the muscles of the tongue, neck, trunk, face, and eyes. Clinically, dystonic reactions may present as a torticollis (neck muscles), hyperextension of the trunk, facial grimacing or tics, dysphagia, or an oculogyric crisis (extraocular muscles). These reactions appear suddenly and generally occur within the first 5 days of treatment with an antipsychotic drug. Young males are the group most prone to develop an acute dystonic reaction. Although these reactions can be frightening to the patient, they can be rapidly reversed. Treatment consists of an immediate IM or, preferably, IV injection of one of the antiparkinsonian drugs listed in Table 1.2, and reassuring the patient that the reaction is transient and can be treated rapidly. The patient can then be treated with an oral antiparkinsonian drug for several days until the risk of developing another dystonic reaction diminishes. Treatment with antipsychotics need not be interrupted. However, it is important to keep in mind that another dystonic reaction could develop with a rapid increase in dose. Also, some patients on depot fluphenazine or haloperidol preparations may have recurrent dystonic reactions following each injection.

Drug-Induced Parkinsonism

Drug-induced parkinsonism presents just like idiopathic parkinsonism, except that the "pill-rolling" tremor is less prominent. It generally occurs between 5 and 30 days after the initiation of treatment and is characterized by bradykinesia, rigidity, shuffling gait, masklike facies, drooling, and a variable tremor. It is more common in older patients, paralleling the incidence of idiopathic parkinsonism. At times *akinesia* (an absence or marked decrease in voluntary movement) may be the predominant feature of parkinsonism and, coupled with the masklike facial expression of these patients, can be confused with psychotic withdrawal or depression. Drug-induced parkinsonism may respond to a lowering of the dose of antipsychotic medication or switching to a lower-potency drug. It also generally responds well to oral antiparkinsonian drugs, and treatment with antipsychotic drugs need not be interrupted.

Akathisia

Akathisia is a syndrome characterized by motor restlessness. Clinically, patients describe an inner sense of stimulation and feel as though they "can't sit still." Consequently, they may be observed pacing or fidgeting. It generally occurs between 5 days and 2 months after initiation of treatment and is often misdiagnosed as psychotic agitation. It is the most difficult extrapyramidal syndrome to both diagnose and treat, as it is less responsive to the antiparkinsonian drugs. However, it may respond to a reduction in dose or a switch to another antipsychotic drug. Antianxiety drugs (e.g., diazepam, lorazepam) may be of some benefit, and recently propranolol in low to moderate doses (20 to 80 mg/d) has been shown to be effective. This latter treatment appears to be the most promising. Treatment with antipsychotics need not be interrupted if the akathisia can be adequately controlled with other agents.

Other Neurological Side Effects

"Rabbit" Syndrome or Perioral Tremor

Perioral tremor ("rabbit" syndrome) is so named because of the peculiar movements associated with it. It is a relatively rare, late-appearing side effect that can be seen in chronically treated patients. Although it does not occur until after months or years of treatment with antipsychotic drugs, it appears to be more similar to parkinsonism than tardive dyskinesia. The rate of the perioral tremor is similar to the rate of the "pill-rolling" tremor of parkinsonism, and thus this entity may represent a late, localized variant of parkinsonism. It often responds well to treatment with antiparkinsonian drugs and is generally reversible after the antipsychotic drug has been discontinued.

Tardive Dyskinesia

Tardive dyskinesia is a late-appearing extrapyramidal syndrome manifested by rhythmic, involuntary, persistent movements of the tongue, lips, and facial muscles. Choreoathetoid movements of the limbs (particularly the fingers and toes) and the trunk may also occur. Occasionally the muscles that control breathing or swallowing can be affected. Characteristically, these movements include tongue protrusion, licking or smacking of the lips, gum-chewing movements, facial grimacing, and eye blinking. In their most serious form they can interfere with eating and speaking and in some cases breathing. In general, tardive dyskinesia occurs in patients who have been on moderate-to-high doses of antipsychotics for long periods of time. However, it may occur after only a few months of treatment. Older patients, particularly women, are at greater risk for the development of tardive dyskinesia, but it can occur at any age. Patients with affective disorders appear to be at greater risk than those with schizophrenia for the development of this syndrome. With the exception of clozapine, all of the antipsychotic drugs can produce this disorder, and none appears to be safer than the others in this regard. The incidence of tardive dyskinesia has been reported to be approximately 15% for those patients treated with antipsychotic drugs for one year or more. Tardive dyskinesia may appear at any time (after several months) during the course of antipsychotic drug treatment, but commonly first appears after the medication has been either reduced or stopped. The current hypothesis to explain tardive dyskinesia is based on the concept of denervation hypersensitivity. After the prolonged blockade of postsynaptic dopaminergic receptors caused by the antipsychotic drugs, it is thought that these receptors become hypersensitive (up-regulated) to dopamine. Thus, there is the development of dopaminergic hypersensitivity with a relative reduction in cholinergic activity. At the present time there is no satisfactory treatment for tardive dyskinesia. The antiparkinsonian drugs are of no benefit and will exacerbate the symptoms of this disorder. Paradoxically, increasing the dose of the antipsychotic drug will temporarily suppress the movements. However, this is not a recommended treatment and should only be done as an extreme measure to treat a disabling dyskinesia. If tardive dyskinesia is recognized early enough and the antipsychotic drug is slowly reduced and discontinued, it will often remit. If it has been present for some time, it will often persist despite discontinuing the antipsychotic drug. As the movements are made worse by anxiety or agitation (they disappear with sleep), a benzodiazepine such as diazepam may be of some benefit. Also the dopamine-depleting drug reserpine may be helpful. It has the advantage of having some antipsychotic effect, but side effects of hypotension and depression may limit its use. The key to decreasing the incidence of this syndrome is prevention and early detection. Antipsychotic drugs should be prescribed only for those patients who will truly benefit from them. Regular neurological assessment of patients on antipsychotic drugs should be performed, and periodic attempts to decrease and discontinue the antipsychotic drug should be made.

The risk of developing a syndrome such as tardive dyskinesia, which may not be reversible, and for which there is no effective treatment, underscores the need to obtain informed consent for treatment with antipsychotic drugs. The risks versus the benefits of prolonged treatment (greater than 6 months) with antipsychotic drugs should be thoroughly discussed with the patient, and his or her informed consent for treatment should be obtained and documented in the medical record. This should be done as soon as the patient's condition has improved to the point where he or she is competent to give informed consent for treatment. If the patient is not competent, informed consent should be obtained from a family member or guardian. If a patient should develop tardive dyskinesia, discontinuation of the antipsychotic drug should be strongly considered. However, the clinician must weigh the risk of a worsening in the psychosis against the risk of a worsening of the tardive dyskinesia. Consultation with a colleague knowledgeable in the area of psychopharmacology would be recommended. After receiving input from the physician, the patient or family member should again give informed consent for the proposed plan of treatment. Recent studies give support to the concept that tardive dyskinesia is generally not a progressive disorder. Thus, symptoms of the disorder may not worsen despite continued treatment with antipsychotic drugs.

Neuroleptic Malignant Syndrome

Neuroleptic malignant syndrome (NMS), a potentially fatal complication of antipsychotic drug treatment, is characterized by muscular rigidity, fever, altered consciousness, and autonomic dysfunction. Although originally thought to be quite rare, it has been reported with increasing frequency; the incidence is reported to be about 1%. The mortality rate is approximately 20%. Men are at greater risk than women by about a 2:1 ratio. Over 80% of patients who develop NMS are under 40 years old. It is more commonly seen following treatment with high-potency drugs (e.g., haloperidol, fluphenazine), especially when high doses are used, but has been reported with low-potency agents. Concurrent treatment with lithium appears to increase the risk of developing NMS. It often occurs within 2 weeks of initiating treatment with an antipsychotic or increasing the dose. However, it may occur after months of treatment with a stable dose regimen. Clinically, patients present with a "lead-pipe rigidity," fever (up to 106°F), tachycardia, diaphoresis, and labile blood pressure. Consciousness is decreased and may progress to stupor or coma. Laboratory findings often include a leukocytosis ranging from 15,000 to 30,000 and an elevated creatinine phosphokinase (CPK) up to 15,000 units or higher. However, no specific laboratory test is diagnostic of NMS. Fatalities in NMS are secondary to respiratory failure, renal failure, and cardiovascular collapse.

Respiratory failure may be due to hypoventilation, pulmonary embolus caused by prolonged immobilization, and aspiration pneumonia caused by dysphagia. Renal failure is due to rhabdomyolysis and myoglobinuria. Treatment of NMS consists of prompt discontinuation of the antipsychotic drug and supportive medical care (e.g., antipyretics, cooling blankets, and restoration of fluid and electrolyte imbalance). Ventilation may be required, and the presence of renal failure may necessitate dialysis. The patient should be given nothing by mouth until he or she is alert enough to take fluids orally and dysphagia is no longer present. Antihypertensive drugs may need to be given to control blood pressure, as may antiarrhythmics. Antiembolism stockings may help to avoid thrombophlebitis and subsequent pulmonary emboli. If the diagnosis of NMS is made early enough, the antipsychotic medication promptly discontinued, and supportive medical care instituted, most patients will recover completely without complications. For more-severe cases of NMS, pharmacologic intervention may be helpful. The muscle relaxant dantrolene, in oral doses between 4 and 10 mg/kg/d given in a qid regimen, may be helpful. Also the dopamine agonists bromocriptine (in doses of 2.5 to 20 mg tid) and amantadine (in doses of 100 mg bid) have been reported to be efficacious in reversing the course of NMS. The combination of bromocriptine and dantrolene appears to be especially promising. Benzodiazepines may also be helpful, both in reversing the symptoms of NMS and in helping to control the patient's agitation. The anticholinergic antiparkinsonian drugs may enhance the autonomic instability of NMS and should probably be avoided. As with tardive dyskinesia, early diagnosis is critical in the management of this potentially life-threatening syndrome. Even signs of mild rigidity and a low-grade fever should raise the possibility of NMS for the alert clinician. After recovery from NMS, treatment with an antipsychotic drug may still be required. If this is the case, it would seem reasonable to cautiously begin therapy with a different antipsychotic drug, preferably a low-potency agent.

Agranulocytosis and Leukopenia

Agranulocytosis and leukopenia are seen most commonly with the aliphatic and piperidine phenothiazines, chlorprothixene, and clozapine. Agranulocytosis is a potentially fatal suppression of the granulocyte series of white blood cells, leaving the body vulnerable to develop an overwhelming infection. As noted previously, the relatively high incidence (1% to 2%) of agranulocytosis associated with clozapine delayed its approval in the United States. The incidence of agranulocytosis with the low-potency phenothiazines is less than 0.01%, making this a very rare complication of treatment. It usually occurs within the first 2 or 3 months of treatment and appears to be an idiosyncratic reaction unrelated to dosage. Elderly women are at greater risk to develop agranulocytosis. Because it occurs abruptly, occasional routine monitoring of the white blood cell (WBC) count is of little aid in its detection. Thus it must be suspected by the clinician if a patient develops a sore throat, fever, or cellulitis, and a WBC count should be obtained immediately. Treatment consists of prompt discontinuation of the antipsychotic drug and institution of appropriate antibiotic therapy. Weekly white blood cell counts for patients being treated with clozapine are recommended because of the greater risk with this drug. Leukopenia is more common but much less serious than agranulocytosis. It is often transient and of no clinical significance, but if it persists, the clinician may want to switch to a different antipsychotic drug.

Cholestatic Jaundice

Cholestatic jaundice has become an increasingly rare side effect of the phenothiazines. Chlorpromazine has been the most frequently implicated drug. It appears to be a sensitivity reaction, unrelated to the dose of the drug administered. Most cases develop during the second to fourth weeks of drug treatment. It is generally mild and self-limited, but it does warrant switching to another class of antipsychotic drugs if continued treatment is necessary.

Photosensitivity

Photosensitivity is another side effect most often associated with chlorpromazine and, like other sensitivity reactions, is not dose-related. Patients can get a severe sunburn with minimal exposure to sunlight. It can be prevented by avoiding exposure to ultraviolet light and by using protective sunscreen preparations. If it becomes troublesome, the patient should be switched to another group of phenothiazines (cross-sensitivity is rare) or to another class of antipsychotic drugs.

Metabolic and Endocrine Effects

Delayed ovulation and menstruation, amenorrhea, breast enlargement and tenderness, and galactorrhea have all been reported as side effects of antipsychotic drug administration. Most often these are seen in women who have been treated chronically with antipsychotics. Gynecomastia and impotence may be seen in men. Both sexes may experience decreased libido. These side effects are caused by hyperprolactinemia and altered hypothalamic and pituitary function. They have most often been associated with the low-potency phenothiazines. As noted previously, thioridazine also causes retrograde ejaculation in men as a result of its peripheral α-adrenergic blockade. Amantadine may be helpful in treating those neuroendocrine side effects caused by increased prolactin release (e.g., galactorrhea, gynecomastia, impotence, breast tenderness, and amenorrhea).

Increased appetite and weight gain can be seen with antipsychotic drugs and can be pronounced. These side effects are also more common with the low-potency phenothiazines. Molindone is the only antipsychotic drug that may actually decrease appetite and facilitate weight loss. It should be considered for those patients in whom weight gain is problematic or who are overweight prior to starting treatment.

Because of their effect on hypothalamic function, antipsychotic drugs can affect the body's temperature-regulating mechanism. Clinically, this increases the risk of developing heat stroke in the summer and hypothermia in the winter.

Lowering of the Convulsive Threshold

Although all antipsychotic drugs lower the seizure threshold to some degree, this complication appears to be more of a problem with the low-potency phenothiazines and loxapine. This is a dose-related side effect that calls for caution when antipsychotic drugs are used in epileptic patients. The dosage of anticonvulsants may need to be increased in epileptics who require treatment with antipsychotic drugs.

Skin and Eye Effects

The skin and eye group of side effects has been associated primarily with chlorpromazine and thioridazine. The most serious of these is the degenerative pigmentary retinopathy (retinitis pigmentosa) caused by prolonged use of thioridazine at daily doses exceeding 800 mg/d. This can produce an irreversible loss of visual acuity. Opacities of the cornea and lens due to the deposit of drug substances and pigment have been reported with prolonged high doses of chlorpromazine. These changes can be visualized on slit-lamp examination. They rarely impair vision and gradually disappear after the drug is stopped.

Deposition of pigment in the skin following prolonged high-dose chlorpromazine treatment can result in a bluish-gray discoloration over skin areas exposed to sunlight. Photosensitivity, the most common skin reaction, has been described previously. Maculopapular skin rashes may also occur. They are generally seen between the first and eighth week of treatment and are non-dose-related allergic reactions. They are best handled by discontinuing the offending drug and switching to another class of antipsychotic agent once the rash clears.

USE IN PREGNANCY AND LACTATION

There is no convincing evidence that antipsychotic drugs increase the risk of fetal malformations. However, it is good practice to avoid the use of antipsychotics during pregnancy whenever possible, especially during the first trimester. Whether or not to use an antipsychotic drug during pregnancy requires good clinical judgment on the part of the physician and the informed consent of the patient (or responsible family member). If an antipsychotic drug is to be used during pregnancy, low doses of a high-potency agent (given in divided doses) are recommended. The low-potency drugs (e.g., chlorpromazine, thioridazine) may carry some added risk of teratogenicity and may complicate delivery because of their hypotensive side effects.

Antipsychotic drugs are secreted in breast milk in low levels, and therefore breastfeeding by mothers on antipsychotics should be avoided.

USE IN THE ELDERLY

The elderly are more sensitive to all of the side effects of the antipsychotic drugs. However, the hypotensive, sedative, and anticholinergic side effects of the low-potency drugs may be particularly troublesome for the elderly. Excessive sedation may cause increased confusion and disorientation. Postural hypotension may result in falls and subsequent fractures. Urinary hesitancy and retention may be seen in elderly males with enlarged prostates. Constipation, tachycardia, and blurry near vision may also be more problematic than they would be for a younger patient. In general, treatment with low, divided doses of the higher-potency antipsychotic drugs is recommended for the elderly. These agents do carry a greater risk for extrapyramidal side effects, but have a lower incidence of most of the other side effects. Use of the anticholinergic antiparkinsonian drugs is not recommended in the elderly. In addition to the anticholinergic side effects noted above, the elderly may develop a toxic delirium secondary to the potent anticholinergic effects of these drugs. The elderly brain is exquisitely sensitive to drugs with anticholinergic effects. If extrapyramidal side effects occur, lowering the dose of the drug, switching to another drug, or treatment with amantadine are potential options.

DRUG INTERACTIONS

Because the antipsychotics are often prescribed along with other drugs (especially in the elderly), it is important to know the potential interactions with these other agents. Several clinically significant drug interactions are described here.

1. The central sedative effects of antipsychotics are additive when given with other drugs that have CNS-depressant properties, which include drugs such as alcohol, anesthetics, sedative-hypnotics, antianxiety agents, antihistamines, narcotics, and tricyclic antidepressants. Oversedation can occur when the antipsychotics are combined with any of these agents. This is particularly true with the sedating phenothiazines. In cases where phenothiazines are given with drugs that can depress respiration (narcotics, sedatives), the clinician must be aware of possible potentiation of this effect.

2. The anticholinergic properties of the antipsychotics will likewise be additive to those of other drugs with anticholinergic effects. Drugs in this group include the anticholinergic antiparkinsonian agents, antihistamines, tricyclic antidepressants, and belladonna alkaloids. It is important to note that many illicit "street drugs" contain varying amounts of belladonna alkaloids. A fairly common combination that could lead to severe anticholinergic side effects is one of an antipsychotic drug, an antiparkinsonian agent, and a tricyclic antidepressant. In cases of anticholinergic drug toxicity, the treatment of choice is physostigmine (Antilirium), a cholinesterase inhibitor that crosses the blood-brain barrier.

3. Combinations of antipsychotics having α-adrenergic-blocking properties (e.g., chlorpromazine, thioridazine, chlorprothixene) with antihypertensive drugs such as reserpine, alpha-methyldopa, or propranolol (and other beta-blockers) may have additive effects resulting in a more pronounced degree of hypotension.

4. Chlorpromazine prevents guanethidine (Ismelin), guanadrel (Hylorel), and other postganglionic blocking drugs from reaching their receptor site of action. When given together, the result is a reversal of the antihypertensive effects of guanethidine and guanadrel. Other phenothiazines may have a similar effect to a lesser degree.

5. The effects of cardiac drugs such as quinidine and procainamide may be potentiated by those antipsychotics (thioridazine, chlorpromazine) that have a myocardial depressant effect, resulting in prolonged ventricular repolarization. Thus, the combination of quinidine or digitalis and thioridazine could increase the likelihood of developing a ventricular arrhythmia.

6. Gel-type antacids (e.g., Maalox, Gelusil) have been shown to decrease serum levels of phenothiazines. Apparently the phenothiazine is adsorbed into the gel structure of the antacid, which inhibits its absorption from the gastro-

intestinal tract. To prevent this interaction, antacids should be administered either 2 hours before or 2 hours after phenothiazines are given.

7. Barbiturates induce hepatic microsomal enzymes and therefore increase the metabolism (and lower the plasma levels) of antipsychotic drugs. Carbamazepine (Tegretol) also can decrease the effect of antipsychotic drugs by increasing their metabolism.

8. Studies have shown that tricyclic antidepressants inhibit the metabolism of antipsychotic drugs, thus leading to higher plasma levels of the latter. The reverse also appears to be true, in that antipsychotic drugs inhibit the metabolism of tricyclic antidepressants. Thus, when these drugs are given together (e.g., amitriptyline and perphenazine) they potentiate each other's effect and should be given in lower doses than when administered separately.

9. As one might expect from their mechanism of action, the antipsychotic drugs antagonize the effects of levadopa and amphetamines.

10. When chlorpromazine and propranolol (Inderal) are given together, there is an increase in the plasma levels of both drugs. Propranolol has also been shown to increase plasma levels of thioridazine.

11. The combination of haloperidol and indomethacin (Indocin) has been reported to cause severe drowsiness.

12. The combination of haloperidol and methyldopa (Aldomet) has been reported to cause a transient dementia. Methyldopa acts as a false transmitter for dopamine and thus may enhance the potent dopamine-receptor blocking action of haloperidol.

13. Chlorpromazine and thioridazine may inhibit the metabolism of phenytoin (Dilantin) and thus lead to phenytoin toxicity.

14. When an antipsychotic drug is given concomitantly with lithium, increased neurotoxicity of both drugs can be seen. There is an increased incidence of neuroleptic malignant syndrome when lithium is combined with an antipsychotic drug. However, this combination can be safe and effective, provided that the patient is closely monitored.

CHAPTER 2

Antidepressant Drugs

The first drugs used to treat depression were the amphetamines, which came into use in the late 1930s. These drugs currently are of limited use in the treatment of depressive illness, and they are best thought of as central nervous system (CNS) stimulants rather than as antidepressant drugs. Problems with the development of tolerance and abuse have further curtailed their use in medical practice.

The two main classes of antidepressant drugs used today are the tricyclic antidepressants and the monoamine oxidase (MAO) inhibitors. Imipramine hydrochloride, the first of the tricyclic compounds, was originally developed in search of an antipsychotic of the phenothiazine type. It was found to be ineffective in the treatment of schizophrenia, but had significant antidepressant effects. Since its release in the late 1950s, several other tricyclic antidepressants have also been developed. The antidepressant effect of the MAO inhibitors was also discovered accidentally. In the early 1950s isoniazid and its derivative iproniazid were developed for the treatment of tuberculosis. It was noted that both of these drugs, but especially iproniazid, had mood-elevating effects in patients with tuberculosis. Iproniazid was found to be a potent inhibitor of the enzyme monoamine oxidase, and by 1957 it was introduced into psychiatry for the treatment of depressed patients. Subsequently, other drugs with the capacity to inhibit MAO were developed for the treatment of depression.

More recently, several newer drugs have been developed and marketed for the treatment of depression. These agents are often referred to as "atypical antidepressants" or "second-generation antidepressants" to distinguish them from the tricyclic antidepressants and the MAO inhibitors. These newer drugs have different chemical structures, and some appear to exert their antidepressant effect via different mechanisms than the older agents. They have therefore caused investigators to reexamine current theories about the biochemical basis of depression and the mechanism of action of antidepressant drugs.

CHEMICAL AND PHARMACOLOGIC PROPERTIES

The biochemical basis of depression and the mechanism of action by which antidepressant drugs exert their therapeutic effects are not fully understood at this time. However, much is known regarding the pharmacologic actions of the antidepressant drugs, and various hypotheses have evolved in an attempt to explain their therapeutic properties.

The earliest theory was the amine hypothesis of depression, which states that depression is associated with a relative deficiency of certain amine neurotransmitters in the brain (particularly the catecholamine norepinephrine). Mania, conversely, is associated with an excess or overactivity of norepinephrine. The indoleamine neurotransmitter serotonin also may play a role in depression and mania by modifying the effects of altered norepinephrine neurotransmission. The amine hypothesis was supported by the fact that reserpine, an antihypertensive drug, caused depression in a significant number of patients who were treated with it. Reserpine was found to exert its effect by depleting stores of aminergic neurotransmitters, such as norepinephrine and serotonin. It was also supported by early knowledge of the mechanism of action of the antidepressant drugs. Tricyclic antidepressant drugs block the reuptake of neurotransmitter from the synaptic cleft back into the presynaptic neuron. Thus the concentration of the neurotransmitter in the synapse is increased, correcting any deficiency that may be present. Tricyclic antidepressants have differing effects on the reuptake of norepinephrine and serotonin. For example, desipramine is a potent blocker of norepinephrine reuptake with little effect on serotonin. Amitriptyline, on the other hand, blocks the reuptake of both norepinephrine and serotonin. The mechanism of action of the MAO inhibitors, although different from that of the tricyclic antidepressants, also supported the amine hypothesis. Monoamine oxidase is one of the enzymes involved in the metabolism of norepinephrine and serotonin. The MAO inhibitors work by blocking the intracellular metabolism of these neurotransmitters. Thus, the concentration of available norepinephrine and serotonin within the presynaptic neuron is increased.

More recent findings have challenged the amine hypothesis and have focused more on the chronic effects of antidepressant drugs on receptor sites in the brain. The blockade of neurotransmitter reuptake is an immediate effect of tricyclic antidepressant drugs. However, the antidepressant effect of tricyclics (and other antidepressants) takes 2 to 4 weeks to develop. Also some of the newer (atypical) antidepressants do not block the reuptake of norepinephrine or serotonin. One of the most interesting findings is that various effective treatments for depression all appear to decrease or "down-regulate" β-adrenergic receptors after chronic administration. This is true not only for different antidepressant drugs but also for electroconvulsive therapy. Other receptor changes seen with chronic administration of antidepressant drugs include decreased sensitivity of the presynaptic α_2-adrenergic autoreceptor and increased sensitivity or "up-regulation" of the postsynaptic α-adrenergic receptor. The end result of these receptor changes is the release of more norepinephrine by the neuron and a heightened effect at the α_1 receptor. It also appears that the serotonergic system must be intact in order for down regulation of the β-adrenergic receptors to occur. These findings of changes in receptor sensitivity occur only after chronic (not acute) treatment with antidepressant drugs and parallel the time course required for these drugs to exert their therapeutic effect.

Although these newer findings represent an advance in our understanding of depression and the mechanism of action of the drugs used to treat it, no single theory can provide an adequate explanation for the actions of all an-

ANTIDEPRESSANT DRUGS 35

tidepressant drugs. It does appear that norepinephrine and serotonin play significant roles in regard to the biological basis of depression, but different drugs may act via different mechanisms. Other neurotransmitters (e.g., acetylcholine, histamine, gamma-aminobutyric acid [GABA] may play a role in depression, but further research is needed to establish this.

In this chapter the antidepressant drugs are organized into three categories: tricyclic and tetracyclic drugs, MAO inhibitors, and atypical agents. The chemical and pharmacologic properties of each group will be discussed separately. The recently released tricyclic antidepressant clomipramine (Anafranil) is discussed at the end of this section.

Tricyclic and Tetracyclic Antidepressants

The tricyclic antidepressants are structurally similar to the phenothiazines. The main difference is that the tricyclics have a seven-member central ring compared to the six-member central ring of the phenothiazines. This difference in structure distorts the shape of the tricyclic molecule and gives it different pharmacologic properties than those of the phenothiazines. The tetracyclic antidepressants have a fourth ring, but as their pharmacologic effects are similar to those of the tricyclics, the two types are grouped together in this section. These drugs are fairly well absorbed from the gastrointestinal tract after oral ingestion. Like the phenothiazines, they are lipid-soluble and highly protein-bound. Although some of the tricyclics are available in an injectable form, parenteral use does not appear to hasten their onset of action and may be associated with an increased incidence of cardiovascular side effects. Therefore intramuscular (IM) use of tricyclics is not recommended except in unusual circumstances. Wide variations have been reported in the plasma half-lives of these drugs, but all of them can be assumed to have half-lives of 24 hours or longer. Thus, they can be administered on a once-a-day basis.

These drugs antagonize or block several different types of neurotransmitter receptors. These include the histamine (H_1) receptor, the muscarinic-cholinergic receptor, and the α_1-adrenergic receptor. Antagonism of these receptors is an acute event and apparently not related to the antidepressant activity of these drugs. However, it does appear to be responsible for many of the side effects seen with the tricyclic antidepressants. Blockade of histamine (H_1) receptors causes sedation and possibly weight gain. Blockade of muscarinic-cholinergic receptors causes anticholinergic side effects such as dry mouth, constipation, blurred near vision, sinus tachycardia, and urinary hesitancy or retention. Blockade of α_1-adrenergic receptors causes postural hypotension, reflex tachycardia, and sedation. Tables 2.1, 2.2, and 2.3 rank these drugs according to their relative potencies in blocking these receptors and thus provide a quick reference as to the side-effect profile of each drug. As one can see from the accompanying tables, the more sedating tricyclics also have significant anticholinergic and α-adrenergic blocking effects.

Two properties of the tricyclic antidepressants should be kept in mind during the management of patients. These drugs have a characteristic delay in their clinical onset of action. Although some patients may show significant improvement in 1 week, 2 to 4 weeks at therapeutic doses is generally required before the desired antidepressant effect is seen. The one exception to this rule

Table 2.1. Blockade of Histamine (H₁) Receptors

ANTIDEPRESSANT	RELATIVE POTENCY
Doxepin	Most potent
Trimipramine	
Amitriptyline	
Maprotiline	
Nortriptyline	
Imipramine	
Protriptyline	
Amoxapine	
Desipramine	Least potent

Table 2.2. Blockade of Muscarinic-Cholinergic Receptors

ANTIDEPRESSANT	RELATIVE POTENCY
Amitriptyline	Most potent
Protriptyline	
Trimipramine	
Doxepin	
Imipramine	
Nortriptyline	
Desipramine	
Maprotiline	
Amoxapine	Least potent

Table 2.3. Blockade of Alpha₁ (α₁)-Adrenergic Receptors

ANTIDEPRESSANT	RELATIVE POTENCY
Doxepin	Most potent
Trimipramine	
Amitriptyline	
Amoxapine	
Nortriptyline	
Maprotiline	
Imipramine	
Protriptyline	
Desipramine	Least potent

may be amoxapine, which is claimed to have a more rapid onset of action. Tricyclic antidepressants also have a relatively low margin of safety when taken in overdose. This is of particular concern because these drugs are prescribed for patients who are at an increased risk for suicide. Doses in the range of 1500 to 2000 mg of imipramine (or the equivalent dose of another drug) can be fatal. Lower doses can cause severe toxicity. Because a fatal dose can be approximately ten times the therapeutic dose, caution is required when dispensing these agents to potentially suicidal patients. As a rule of thumb, no more than a week's supply should be given to any patient who is at risk for suicidal behavior.

The metabolism of the tricyclics has important clinical implications. Imipramine and amitryptyline are metabolized by demethylation to desipramine and nortriptyline, respectively. These metabolites are antidepressants in their own right and are marketed as such. Imipramine and amitriptyline are tertiary amines, while desipramine and nortriptyline are secondary amines. In general, the demethylated metabolites (secondary amines) are less sedating and have fewer anticholinergic effects than the tertiary amines. Another difference is that the secondary amines preferentially block the reuptake of norepinephrine, while the tertiary amines block the reuptake of both norepinephrine and serotonin. The proportion of parent compound to demethylated metabolite varies considerably from patient to patient, apparently because of genetic differences in the way these drugs are metabolized. In general, imipramine is more rapidly metabolized to desipramine, producing a higher proportion of the metabolite to the parent drug. In contrast, amitriptyline is more slowly metabolized to nortriptyline, resulting in a higher proportion of the parent drug to the metabolite.

More recently it has been possible to measure plasma levels of tricyclic antidepressants. The clinical use of plasma levels in monitoring treatment with tricyclics has taken on added importance, but effective levels for all tricyclics have not been established. Plasma levels of tricyclics may vary by anywhere from 10-fold to 30-fold in patients receiving a single fixed dose of drug. This finding highlights the marked difference in absorption and metabolism of these drugs among individual patients and stresses the need for flexible clinical dose regimens to meet individual patient requirements. At the present time there are good data correlating plasma level and clinical response for three of the tricyclics. Studies with nortriptyline have shown an effective therapeutic range to be between 50 and 150 ng/mL. Levels below *or* above this range are associated with a poor clinical response. This type of response pattern has been referred to as the "therapeutic window" concept. There is a curvilinear relationship between clinical response and plasma nortriptyline levels. The correlation between plasma level and clinical response for imipramine and desipramine is linear (i.e., the higher the serum level, the better the response). However, excessively high serum levels would be associated with toxicity. For imipramine, plasma levels of imipramine plus desipramine between 200 and 300 ng/mL have been associated with a good clinical response. For desipramine, plasma levels between 100 and 250 ng/mL have been associated with a good clinical response.

When using plasma levels of tricyclics clinically, it is important to keep a few points in mind. First, these levels have been established in patients with major depression. For other indications, including less severe depressions, there is no well-established relationship between tricyclic antidepressant plasma levels and clinical response. Plasma levels should be determined from blood samples drawn 12 hours after the patient's last dose in order to reflect trough values. Also, plasma levels will be most accurate when drawn after "steady-state" conditions have been reached, that is, when a specific dose of the drug given over several days produces a consistent blood level. The "steady state" is reached after approximately five times the half-life of the drug. For the tricyclics, this period is about 5 to 7 days. Finally, these plasma levels are technically difficult assays to do, and it is important to have them done by a reliable clinical laboratory.

The tricyclic antidepressants have several effects on sleep. They significantly decrease rapid-eye-movement (REM) sleep, increase stage 4 sleep, and decrease the number of awakenings. The ability of a tricyclic to suppress the onset of REM sleep early on in treatment may be a predictor of an eventual positive clinical response.

The following sections discuss the important characteristics of each of the tricyclic and tetracyclic drugs.

$$CHCH_2CH_2N(CH_3)_2$$

Amitriptyline

Amitriptyline is the most anticholinergic of all the tricyclics. It is over ten times as potent as desipramine in terms of anticholinergic activity. Along with doxepin and trimipramine, it is also one of the most sedative. Because of its strong anticholinergic side effects, it is often tolerated poorly by the elderly.

The elderly are exquisitely sensitive to the CNS anticholinergic effects of amitriptyline and may develop a toxic delirium similar to atropine toxicity. This is manifested by disorientation, confusion, agitation, recent memory loss, and visual hallucinations. Because of its sedative properties, amitriptyline is often used for those depressions in which anxiety or agitation and insomnia are prominent symptoms. This tricyclic is also effective in the treatment of some chronic pain syndromes. It is the only tricyclic marketed in combination preparations. The amitriptyline-perphenazine combination (Triavil, Etrafon) was discussed in the previous chapter. Amitriptyline is also marketed in combination with the benzodiazepine chlordiazepoxide. The trade name for this preparation is Limbitrol, and it is available in two strengths (one contains 5 mg of chlordiazepoxide and 12.5 mg of amitriptyline; the other contains 10 mg of chlordiazepoxide and 25 mg of amitriptyline). This combination may offer some benefit over amitriptyline alone for those depressions accompanied by a significant degree of anxiety, especially during the first week of treatment. However, amitriptyline alone may be adequate treatment because of its marked sedating properties. Another use for such a combination would be in patients who report overstimulation, restlessness, jitteriness, or insomnia on a tricyclic alone. Should the need to use such a combination arise, the drugs should initially be prescribed separately to allow for better titration of dose. Once a fixed regimen has been established, the combination product may be used. Combinations of other tricyclics and benzodiazepines may also be effective, although none are marketed as such. The advantage of this combination over that of a tricyclic and an antipsychotic (e.g., amitriptyline and perphenazine) is that there is no risk of developing tardive dyskinesia.

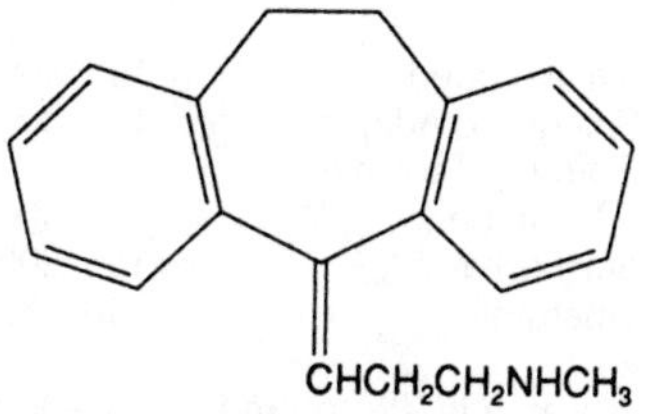

CHCH₂CH₂NHCH₃

Nortriptyline

Nortriptyline is the demethylated metabolite of amitriptyline. It is significantly less sedative and less anticholinergic than the parent drug. It is more potent than amitriptyline on a milligram-per-milligram basis and the upper dose limit is less (see Table 2.4). Studies have shown that nortriptyline produces less postural hypotension than other drugs in this class. Thus it is one of the preferred drugs for use in the elderly and other patients who are prone to develop this side effect. Nortriptyline has also been shown to be effective in poststroke depressions. It is the only tricyclic with a well-defined plasma level "therapeutic window" (50 to 150 ng/mL) response pattern.

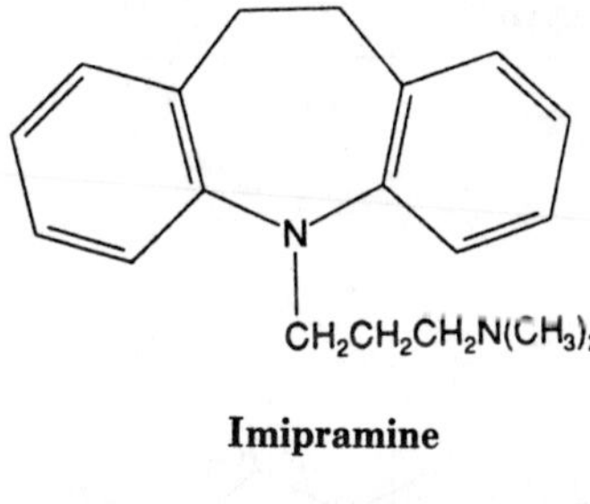

CH₂CH₂CH₂N(CH₃)₂

Imipramine

Imipramine is intermediate in its sedative and anticholinergic properties. It is the oldest tricyclic and has been used more extensively for other indications (e.g., panic disorder, enuresis, attention deficit disorder with hyperactivity) than the other drugs in this class. It is marketed in two forms (imipramine hydrochloride and imipramine pamoate), which are equally efficacious.

Desipramine is the demethylated metabolite of imipramine. It is one of the least anticholinergic of the drugs in this class and therefore useful for those patients in whom anticholinergic side effects might prove troublesome (e.g.,

Table 2.4. Approximate Daily Dose Ranges of Antidepressant Drugs

GENERIC NAME	TRADE NAME	USUAL DAILY DOSE RANGE (mg/d) INPATIENT	OUTPATIENT OR MAINTENANCE
Tricyclic antidepressants			
Tertiary amines			
Amitriptyline*	Elavil, Endep	150–300	50–150
Doxepin*	Sinequan, Adapin	150–300	50–150
Imipramine*	Tofranil, Tofranil-PM, Janimine	150–300	50–150
Trimipramine	Surmontil	150–300	50–150
Clomipramine	Anafranil	150–250	50–150
Secondary amines			
Desipramine*	Norpramin, Pertofrane	150–300	50–150
Nortriptyline	Aventyl, Pamelor	75–150	25–100
Protriptyline	Vivactil	30–60	10–30
Tetracyclic antidepressants			
Amoxapine	Asendin	150–450	75–200
Maprotiline*	Ludiomil	150–225	50–150
Monoamine oxidase inhibitors			
Hydrazines			
Isocarboxazid	Marplan	20–50	10–30
Phenelzine	Nardil	45–90	30–60
Nonhydrazine			
Tranylcypromine	Parnate	20–50	10–30
Atypical antidepressants			
Bupropion	Wellbutrin	200–450	100–300
Fluoxetine	Prozac	40–80	20–40
Trazodone*	Desyrel	200–600	100–400

*Also available generically.

Desipramine

elderly patients or patients with prostatic hypertrophy). It also tends to produce a minimal amount of sedation. Desipramine is a potent blocker of norepinephrine reuptake.

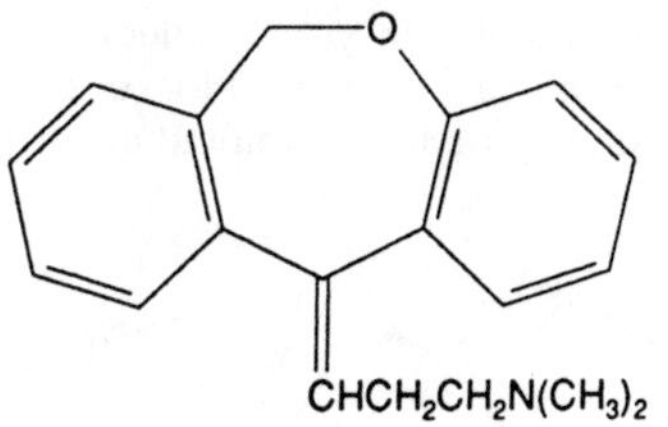

$\overset{|}{C}HCH_2CH_2N(CH_3)_2$

Doxepin

Doxepin is strongly sedating and high in its anticholinergic effects. It is a relatively weak inhibitor of neurotransmitter reuptake and felt by some to be less potent than the other drugs in this class. Studies have shown doxepin to be effective in the treatment of peptic ulcer disease, having comparable effects to cimetidine (Tagamet). This effect is due to doxepin's ability to block the histamine H_2 receptor, which mediates the secretion of gastric acid.

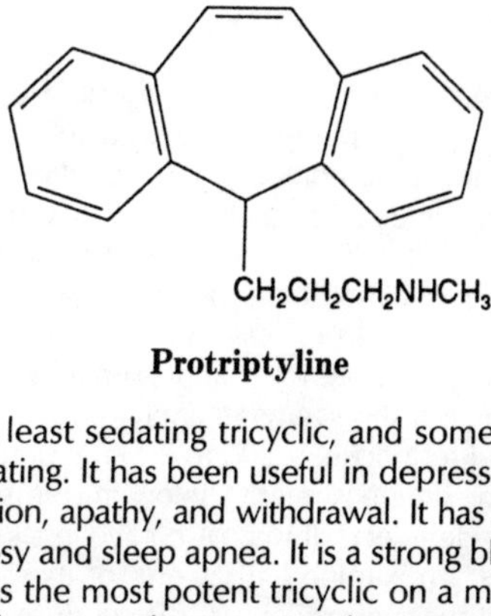

$CH_2CH_2CH_2NHCH_3$

Protriptyline

Protriptyline is the least sedating tricyclic, and some clinicians feel that it may in fact be stimulating. It has been useful in depressions characterized by psychomotor retardation, apathy, and withdrawal. It has also been used in the treatment of narcolepsy and sleep apnea. It is a strong blocker of norepinephrine reuptake, and it is the most potent tricyclic on a milligram-per-milligram basis (approximately five times the potency of amitriptyline and imipramine). It also has the longest elimination half-life of any tricyclic (3 to 5 days) and thus can be particularly problematic when taken In overdose. Anticholinergic side effects tend to be intermediate with protriptyline.

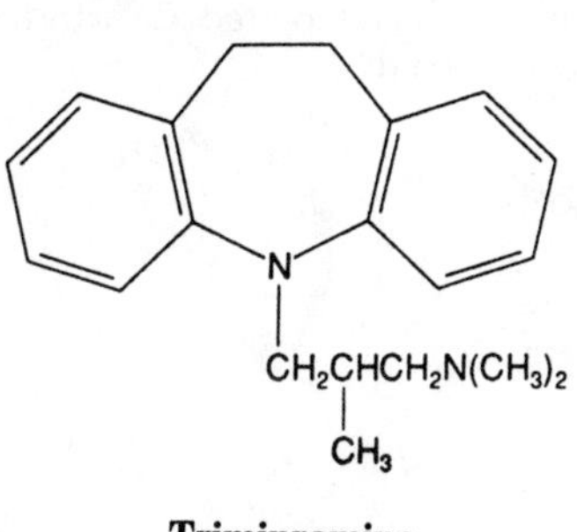

$CH_2\overset{|}{C}HCH_2N(CH_3)_2$
$\overset{|}{C}H_3$

Trimipramine

Trimipramine, a tertiary amine tricyclic antidepressant, is strongly sedating and anticholinergic. It is a relatively weak blocker of neurotransmitter reuptake. Like doxepin and amitriptyline, trimipramine also has potent antihistaminic effects.

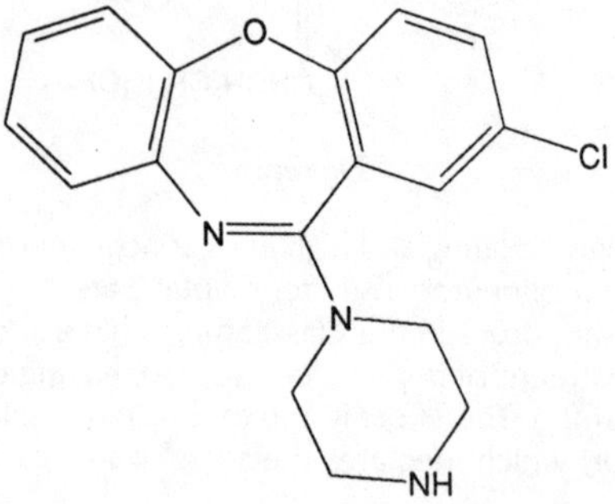

Amoxapine

Amoxapine is a metabolite of the antipsychotic drug loxapine. It is a relatively potent blocker of norepinephrine reuptake. Its major metabolite in humans, 8-hydroxyamoxapine, inhibits the reuptake of serotonin as well as norepinephrine. Amoxapine has a half-life of approximately 8 hours, while 8-hydroxyamoxapine has a half-life of 30 hours. Amoxapine has been claimed to have an earlier onset of action than the other drugs in this class, with most patients responding in 2 weeks or less. However, these reports require further validation. Its milligram potency is approximately one half that of imipramine and amitriptyline, but this seems to apply more at the lower dose range. Most patients respond to a dose of 200 to 300 mg/d, but some require in excess of 300 mg/d. Amoxapine is relatively low in terms of producing anticholinergic and sedative side effects. It may also have less cardiotoxicity. The most interesting feature of amoxapine is that one of its metabolites, 7-hydroxyamoxapine, blocks dopamine receptors. Thus amoxapine is the only antidepressant having neuroleptic (antipsychotic) activity. This may make it more effective in treating depressions with psychotic features, but it also exposes patients to the risks associated with antipsychotic drugs. Tardive dyskinesia is a potential complication with amoxapine, and at least one case of neuroleptic malignant syndrome has been reported. Galactorrhea and akathisia have been more frequently observed.

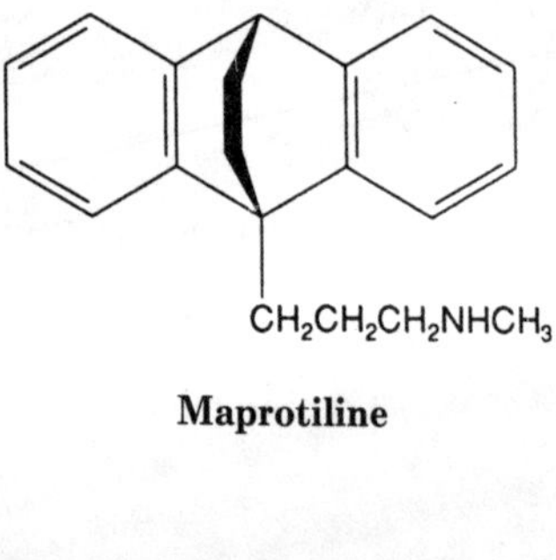

$CH_2CH_2CH_2NHCH_3$

Maprotiline

Maprotiline, as noted in the diagram, has a bridge across the central ring, giving it a three-dimensional structure. This change is responsible for its being called a tetracyclic, but its pharmacologic effects are similar to those of the tricyclics. Maprotiline is a secondary amine and a selective blocker of norepinephrine reuptake. It has virtually no effect on serotonin. Its serum half-life is approximately 48 hours, and steady-state levels are reached after 7 to 10 days of treatment. Maprotiline is as effective as the tricyclics and MAO inhibitors in the treatment of depression, with the typical lag period of 2 to 4 weeks of treatment necessary to achieve a significant therapeutic effect. It produces a moderate degree of sedation and a relatively low incidence of anticholinergic side effects. Maprotiline has also been reported to produce less severe cardiotoxic effects than amitriptyline or imipramine. The most troublesome problem with this drug is that it appears more likely to lower the seizure threshold and induce convulsions than the other antidepressants. This is especially true at doses above 200 mg/d and when the dose of the drug is rapidly increased. Because of maprotiline's higher risk for inducing seizures, the manufacturer recommends a maximum daily dose of 225 mg/d. Maintenance treatment with maprotiline should be at doses of 200 mg/d or less. This drug is contraindicated in patients with a previous history of seizure disorder.

MAO Inhibitors

The MAO inhibitors have not enjoyed the more widespread use of the tricyclic antidepressants in the treatment of depression. Past problems with toxicity and side effects have caused many clinicians to be wary of their use. Iproniazid (Marsilid), one of the early MAO inhibitors, was withdrawn from the market because of severe liver toxicity. Other drugs in this class were removed from the market because of limited efficacy in controlled trials. The potential risk of developing a hypertensive crisis with the use of these drugs remains an important concern.

However, more recently, the role of the MAO inhibitors has been better defined. Although not the treatment of choice for episodes of major depression, they may be useful for those depressions refractory to the tricyclic/tetracyclic or atypical antidepressants. MAO inhibitors have also been found to be effective in the treatment of panic disorder, phobic disorders, and "atypical depressions." These latter depressions are characterized by anxiety, somatic complaints, fatigue hypersomnia, phobias and obsessive symptoms. More recent controlled studies have documented the efficacy of the MAO inhibitors for these conditions.

There are only three MAO inhibitors available for use in psychiatric disorders: isocarboxazid, phenelzine, and tranylcypromine.

The MAO inhibitors can be divided into two classes, hydrazines and nonhydrazines. Isocarboxazid and phenelzine are hydrazine derivatives, while tranylcypromine is a nonhydrazine derivative. The hydrazines carry a greater risk of hepatotoxicity than tranylcypromine, with phenelzine being less hepatotoxic than isocarboxazid. These drugs have minimal, if any, sedative and anticholinergic effects, in contrast to the tricyclic and tetracyclic antidepressants. They also do not produce the cardiotoxic effects sometimes associated with the latter drugs. They may produce unwanted stimulation, especially tranylcypromine. However, the most common side effect of MAO inhibitors is postural hypotension. To obtain an antidepressant effect with these drugs, platelet MAO activity must be about 85% inhibited. The use of too low a dose of these drugs appears to have been responsible for their lack of efficacy in earlier controlled studies. Like the tricyclics and tetracyclics, a 2- to 4-week treatment period is generally required to achieve an optimal antidepressant effect, although tranylcypromine has been reported to produce a more rapid response. Another feature these drugs share with the tricyclics and tetracyclics is their narrow therapeutic index. A 7- to 10-day supply of a MAO inhibitor taken in overdose could be fatal. Thus, the same precautions apply when dealing with potentially suicidal patients.

The MAO inhibitors are readily absorbed after oral administration and produce maximal inhibition of MAO in 5 to 10 days. Phenelzine and isocarboxazid produce an "irreversible" enzyme inhibition, in that it takes approximately 2 weeks (or longer) to recover MAO activity after these drugs are discontinued. With tranylcypromine, however, MAO activity may return in from 7 to 10 days after the drug is stopped. Because of this long-lasting effect on MAO, these drugs can be administered on a once-a-day basis. Monoamine oxidase is a widely distributed enzyme and is responsible for the breakdown of other amines in addition to norepinephrine and serotonin. Epinepherine, dopamine, tyramine, and tryptamine are all metabolized by MAO. Thus, the MAO inhibitors cause an increase in CNS levels of all these amines. Tyramine is a pressor amine and has been implicated as the causative agent in the production of hypertensive crises. These crises have occurred when patients taking MAO inhibitors have ingested foods containing tyramine. Although these reactions are rare, they can be fatal secondary to intracranial hemorrhage. Thus, all patients taking MAO inhibitors must avoid tyramine-containing foods. Also, medications containing sympathomimetic agents must be avoided. These include decongestants (commonly found in cold and sinus preparations) and amphetamines (often a component of diet pills). Caffeine-containing beverages and chocolate should be used only in moderation because of their sympathomimetic effects. A list of foods and drugs to avoid with MAO inhibitors is presented in Table 2.5.

Assuming that an appropriate diet is adhered to, the clinician has to be observant for signs of the more common side effect of postural (orthostatic) hypotension. Symptoms of dizziness and lightheadedness occur in a significant percentage of patients treated with MAO inhibitors. One MAO inhibitor, pargyline (Eutonyl), is actually marketed as an antihypertensive drug. This agent may also have some antidepressant effect, but it is generally not considered as effective as the other MAO inhibitors.

Current research in this area has centered around the development of selective MAO inhibitors that may be less likely to be associated with the development of hypertensive crises. There are two different types of monoamine oxidase, MAO-A and MAO-B. Phenelzine, isocarboxazid, and tranylcypromine are all nonselective MAO inhibitors in that they inhibit both MAO-A and MAO-B. Inhibition of MAO-A appears to be necessary for the antidepressant activity of these drugs. Drugs that are selective for MAO-B may offer greater safety, as intestinal monoamine oxidase is not inhibited by MAO-B type inhibitors. Thus tyramine could be broken down in the gut, and the risk of developing a hypertensive crisis would be less likely. Pargyline and selegiline (Eldepryl;

**Table 2.5. Foods and Drugs to Be Avoided
with Monoamine Oxidase Inhibitors**

Foods

Aged cheeses (cottage cheese, cream cheese, and American processed cheese are permitted).

Beer and red wine (other alcoholic drinks permitted *in moderation only*)

Broad-bean pods (fava or Italian green beans)

Pickled herring, sardines, and anchovies

Yeast extracts (e.g., brewer's yeast, Marmite, Bovril)

Fermented sausages (salami, pepperoni, summer sausage, bologna)

Canned figs

Banana skins (bananas permitted if not overripe)

Any non-fresh, fermented, or preserved liver, meat, or fish product

Yogurt and sour cream (permitted in moderation)

Chocolate (permitted in moderation)

Caffeinated beverages (coffee, tea, colas, cocoa permitted in moderation)

(In general, fresh food or freshly prepared foods that have been frozen or canned can be safely consumed.)

Drugs

Decongestants (e.g., phenylpropanolamine, pseudoephedrine), either alone or as contained in cold preparations, cough medicines, or allergy preparations

Amphetamines and other stimulants

Meperidine (Demerol)

Dental anesthetics containing epinephrine

L-dopa

Cocaine

L-deprenyl) are MAO-B type inhibitors. Selegiline appears to be safer but less effective than the current MAO inhibitors in use. This drug was recently released for the adjunctive treatment (along with levodopa/carbidopa) of Parkinson's disease.

The characteristics of the three MAO inhibitors currently used in the treatment of psychiatric disorders are discussed in the following sections.

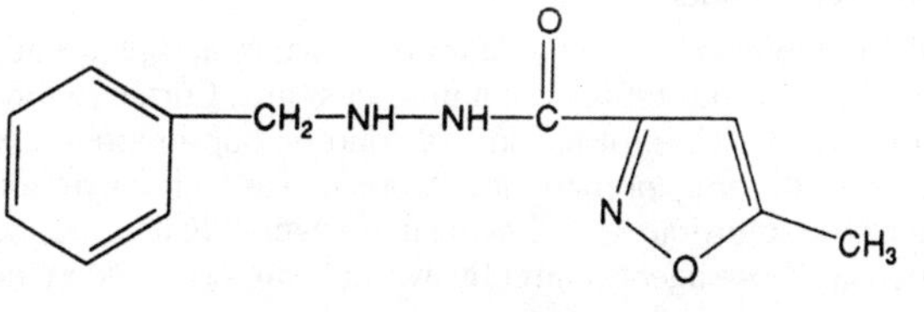

Isocarboxazid

Isocarboxazid is not as frequently prescribed as the other MAO inhibitors. There is some feeling that it may be less effective than phenelzine and tranylcypromine, and it also carries a greater risk of hepatotoxicity. However, it does appear to produce less orthostatic hypotension than phenelzine.

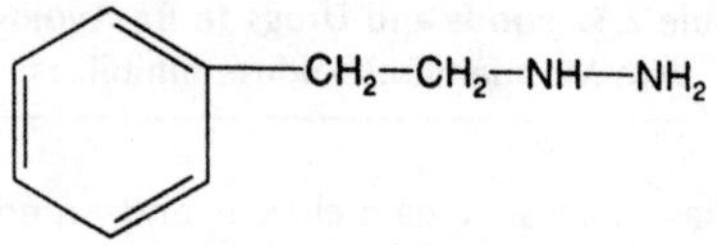

$$\text{(benzene ring)}-CH_2-CH_2-NH-NH_2$$

Phenelzine

Phenelzine has been the most extensively studied and is the most widely used MAO inhibitor. Studies have shown it to be effective in the treatment of atypical depression, panic disorder, and phobic disorders. A dose of 60 mg/d has been reported to produce 85% inhibition of platelet MAO, the level felt to be necessary for an antidepressant effect. Some patients will report mild-to-moderate sedation with phenelzine, while others find it to be stimulating. It appears to be especially useful for depressions with anxious, phobic, or obsessional features.

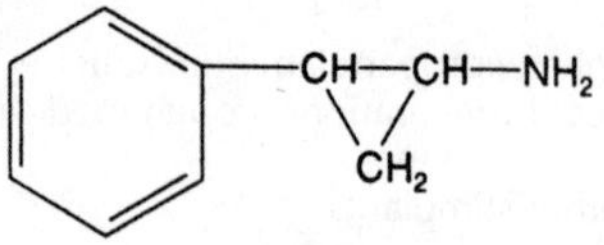

$$\text{(benzene ring)}-CH-CH-NH_2$$
$$\quad\quad\quad\quad | \quad\quad |$$
$$\quad\quad\quad\quad CH_2$$

Tranylcypromine

Tranylcypromine's structure resembles that of the amphetamines, and this property may be responsible for its reported stimulant effect. Because of this effect, it may produce a quicker antidepressant response than phenelzine or isocarboxazid. Tranylcypromine is more potent than phenelzine on a milligram-per-milligram basis. It appears to produce less postural hypotension than phenelzine, but it has more often been associated with the development of hypertensive crises. This drug may be particularly useful for depressions characterized by withdrawal and anergy.

Atypical Antidepressants

Atypical antidepressants have a different structure and pharmacologic profile than the tricyclic and tetracyclic antidepressants. Currently three drugs in this category are available for use in this country: bupropion, fluoxetine, and trazodone. A fourth drug, nomifensine (Merital), was withdrawn from the market by the manufacturer in 1986 because of several deaths secondary to hemolytic anemia. Those agents currently available are discussed in the following sections.

Bupropion is a recently released antidepressant with a unique chemical structure. It is a "unicyclic" belonging to the aminoketone chemical class. It does not block the reuptake of norepinephrine or serotonin to any significant degree, and it does not inhibit monoamine oxidase. At relatively high doses, it is a weak blocker of dopamine reuptake. However, because this effect occurs at doses greater than those required for its antidepressant effect,

Bupropion

it does not appear to be responsible for bupropion's mechanism of action. At the present time the biochemical mechanism of bupropion's antidepressant effect is unknown. Bupropion is well absorbed after oral administration, and peak plasma levels are obtained within 2 hours. The elimination half-life of bupropion is 10 to 14 hours, although this may vary considerably among patients. There are three major metabolites of bupropion, some of which may be active. The average half-lives of the metabolites are longer than that of the parent drug. In controlled clinical trials, bupropion has been shown to have an antidepressant effect similar to that of the standard antidepressant drugs. Interestingly, it does not appear to be effective in the treatment of panic disorder, but may exert a prophylactic effect for bipolar illness. Like the other antidepressant drugs, bupropion requires 2 to 4 weeks of treatment for its antidepressant effect to occur. As one might expect from its structure, bupropion has a distinctly different side-effect profile than the tricyclic and tetracyclic drugs. It has minimal anticholinergic and antihistaminic effects. It rarely causes orthostatic hypotension and has no clinically significant effect on cardiac conduction. Bupropion generally does not cause weight gain and is often associated with a slight weight loss. Oversedation is also not common with this drug. The main side effects that have been associated with bupropion include overstimulation, agitation, insomnia, dizziness, headache, dry mouth, nausea, and tremor. Several of these side effects are secondary to bupropion's mild stimulant properties. Because of these properties, it is generally best not to give bupropion at bedtime. Bupropion has been associated with a 0.4% incidence of generalized seizures, slightly higher than that for other antidepressants. In February 1986, the drug was withdrawn from the market by the manufacturer after the occurrence of seizures in several bulimic patients. However, further studies have shown that the induction of seizures by bupropion is not excessive in comparison with other antidepressants as long as certain precautions are taken. To reduce the risk of developing seizures with bupropion, it is recommended that the total daily dose not exceed 450 mg and that no more than 150 mg be given as a single dose. A gradual increase in the dose of bupropion will also help to minimize the risk of seizure induction. At the present time the manufacturer states that the drug is contraindicated in patients with a seizure disorder and in patients with a current or prior diagnosis of bulimia or anorexia nervosa. Extreme caution should be used when prescribing bupropion for any patient with a predisposition to developing a seizure (e.g., history of significant head trauma). In summary, bupropion appears to be an effective antidepressant drug with a favorable side-effect profile. If proper precautions are taken, the risk of seizures can be kept to an incidence not much greater than that for other antidepressants.

$$F_3C-\langle\text{ring}\rangle-O-CH-CH_2CH_2NHCH_3 \cdot HCl$$

Fluoxetine

Fluoxetine was released for use in this country in January 1988 and has quickly become one of the most frequently prescribed antidepressant drugs. It is chemically unrelated to the other available antidepressants and is sometimes referred to as a "bicyclic" as it possesses two rings. Fluoxetine is a potent and specific inhibitor of serotonin reuptake with little effect on norepinephrine and dopamine. It is much more potent in its effect on serotonin than amitriptyline or doxepin. The selective action on serotonin reuptake differentiates it from the other antidepressants. It is also a very weak blocker of histamine (H_1) receptors, muscarinic-cholinergic receptors, and α_1-adrenergic receptors. Fluoxetine is well absorbed after oral administration, reaching peak plasma levels 6 to 8 hours after a single dose. It is a long-acting drug with an elimination half-life of 2 to 3 days. Its active metabolite, norfluoxetine, is also a potent and selective inhibitor of serotonin reuptake and has a half-life of 7 to 9 days.

Controlled clinical trials have shown fluoxetine to be more effective than placebo and as effective as amitriptyline, imipramine, and doxepin in the treatment of major depression in an outpatient population. As with the other antidepressants, 2 to 4 weeks of treatment with fluoxetine are generally required for an antidepressant effect to occur. Fluoxetine has also been reported to be effective in the treatment of obsessive compulsive disorder (OCD). Although not yet approved for use in this disorder, it appears to hold much promise as an effective treatment. Other possible uses for fluoxetine include the treatment of obesity, alcoholism, bulimia, chronic pain, and panic disorder. Its specific and potent effect on serotonin reuptake appears to be related to its effectiveness in the treatment of disorders of impulse control.

In comparison with the tricyclic and tetracyclic antidepressants, fluoxetine generally has a more favorable (milder) side-effect profile. It produces a low incidence of anticholinergic side effects and postural hypotension. Drowsiness and oversedation are also less common with fluoxetine. It produces no clinically significant electrocardiogram (ECG) changes and is not associated with tachycardia. Studies have shown a slight decrease in heart rate in patients treated with fluoxetine. It has not been associated with seizure induction when taken in therapeutic doses and also appears to be relatively safe when taken in an overdose. In contrast to most tricyclic and tetracyclic drugs, which have been associated with weight gain, fluoxetine actually appears to facilitate weight loss. The main side effects associated with fluoxetine are nausea, nervousness and anxiety, insomnia, headache, diarrhea, anorexia, drowsiness, tremor, and excessive sweating. These side effects are generally mild, occur early in treatment, and tend to decrease over time. About 4% of patients treated with fluoxetine in clinical trials developed a rash and/or urticaria. Like other antidepressants, fluoxetine may precipitate manic or hypomanic episodes in bipolar depressed patients. Fluoxetine should not be used concomitantly with MAO inhibitors. A patient should be off a MAO inhibitor for at least 14 days before initiation of treatment with fluoxetine. If switching from fluoxetine to a MAO inhibitor, a 5-week "washout period" is recommended before starting treatment with the MAO inhibitor, because of fluoxetine's long half-life and the long half-life of its active metabolite.

Treatment with fluoxetine should be initiated with a dose of 20 mg/d. This dose is given in the morning because of fluoxetine's tendency to produce insomnia. Because of fluoxetine's long half-life, 2 to 4 weeks are required to reach steady-state plasma concentrations. Dose increases should be very gradual with this drug. Doses higher than 20 mg/d should be given on a twice-a-day regimen (e.g., morning and noon). The maximum daily recommended dose for fluoxetine is 80 mg. Most depressed patients appear to respond to 20 to 40 mg/d of fluoxetine, but doses in the range of 60 to 80 mg/d appear to be required in the treatment of OCD.

In summary, fluoxetine appears to be as effective as the standard antidepressants in the treatment of depression. Its mild side-effect profile, as compared with the tricyclic and tetracyclic antidepressants, makes it an appropriate choice for patients who cannot tolerate the latter drugs. In particular, its low incidence of anticholinergic and cardiovascular side effects makes it a good choice for the treatment of the elderly depressed patient. Its relative safety in overdose, lack of propensity to induce seizures, and absence of weight gain are additional favorable qualities. Fluoxetine may be efficacious in the treatment of resistant depressions, and at least one study has found it superior to a tricyclic antidepressant for the treatment of atypical depression.

There have been recent reports of depressed patients developing suicidal ideation after treatment with fluoxetine was initiated. A review of the subject found that a small percentage of patients report suicidal ideation after the onset of treatment with antidepressant drugs. This effect does not appear to be significantly higher with fluoxetine than with other antidepressants. Because of its activating and stimulating properties, fluoxetine could theoretically activate latent suicidal thoughts.

Trazodone is a triazolopyridine derivative, chemically unrelated to the tricyclic/tetracyclic and other currently marketed antidepressants. It is a serotonin reuptake inhibitor and also has both agonist and antagonist effects on serotonin receptors in the CNS. It is a weak blocker of histamine (H_1) receptors and muscarinic-cholinergic receptors. However, it does have significant α-adrenergic receptor blocking effects. Trazodone is rapidly absorbed after oral administration, reaching peak plasma levels in 0.5 to 2 hours. It is absorbed

Trazodone

faster and attains higher blood levels when given on an empty stomach. It has a relatively short half-life of approximately 10 hours.

Multiple controlled studies have found trazodone to be as effective as the tricyclics in the treatment of depression. It has a delay in its onset of action similar to that of the other antidepressants. The therapeutic dose range is from 50 mg (in some elderly patients) to 600 mg/d, with most patients responding to 150 to 300 mg/d. It is reported to be approximately one half the milligram potency of imipramine. Some clinicians have proposed that trazodone has a therapeutic window similar to nortriptyline. Thus, doses and plasma levels that are too high may be associated with a poor response.

As trazodone is highly sedating, some clinicians find it useful for those depressions in which anxiety and insomnia are prominent features. In addition to excessive sedation, other commonly seen side effects include nausea, postural hypotension with secondary dizziness and fainting, headache, and dry mouth. Although trazodone has minimal anticholinergic effects, it causes dry mouth because of its effect on norepinephrine activity. Nausea can be diminished by giving it after meals, as can dizziness and headache. Trazodone has minimal effects on cardiac-conduction, but patients with preexisting ventricular irritability can develop ventricular ectopic beats. A side effect unique to trazodone is the occurrence of priapism. Although this is quite rare, approximately one third of the cases reported have required surgical intervention. If not effectively treated, priapism may result in permanent impotence. Because of this, some clinicians are hesitant to prescribe trazodone for men. Male patients should be instructed to discontinue the drug immediately and consult their physician should they experience any symptoms suggestive of priapism (i.e., prolonged or inappropriate erections). Trazodone does not appear to exacerbate psychotic symptoms when given to patients with schizophrenia or schizoaffective disorder. It also appears to be less likely than the tricyclic antidepressants to precipitate manic episodes. As with fluoxetine, trazodone has not been associated with seizure induction and is relatively safe when taken in an overdose.

In summary, trazodone is an effective antidepressant drug with significant sedating properties. Although not as potent as the tricyclic antidepressants or MAO inhibitors, it may be especially useful for patients with mild to moderate depression characterized by significant anxiety or insomnia.

Recently Released Antidepressant

Although there are several promising antidepressants in the investigational category, clomipramine (Anafranil) was released for use in early 1990 and is discussed here. It is the only drug currently approved for the treatment of OCD.

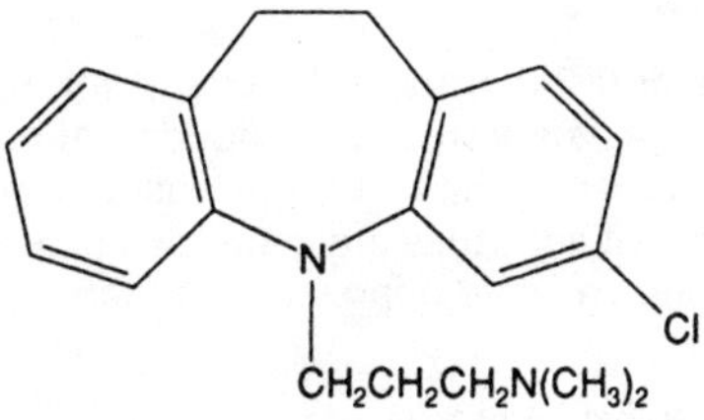

$CH_2CH_2CH_2N(CH_3)_2$

Clomipramine

Clomipramine is a tricyclic antidepressant that is in common use in Europe and Canada. It differs from imipramine only in having a chlorine atom at the 3-position of the tricyclic structure. Of all the tricyclics it is the most potent blocker of serotonin reuptake. However, its metabolite, desmethyl clomipramine, blocks the reuptake of both norepinephrine and serotonin. Clomipramine has been shown to be effective in the treatment of OCD, presumably secondary to its effect on serotonin. Its effectiveness in the treatment of OCD appears to be independent of its antidepressant activity. It is the only tricyclic antidepressant found to be effective in the treatment of OCD in controlled trials. The dose range for clomipramine is similar to that for imipramine and amitriptyline, except that the recommended upper dose limit is 250 mg/d because of a higher incidence of seizures with this tricyclic. Improvement in the symptoms of OCD occurs gradually with clomipramine, with 2 or more months of treatment needed to obtain optimal benefit from the drug. The main side effects seen with clomipramine are oversedation, anticholinergic effects, tremor, and sexual dysfunction.

INDICATIONS FOR USE

Major Depression, Single Episode or Recurrent

Major depression is the primary indication for the use of antidepressant drugs. A major depressive episode is characterized by depressed mood, markedly diminished interest or pleasure in most activities, insomnia or hypersomnia, decrease or increase in appetite or significant weight loss or weight gain, psychomotor agitation or retardation, fatigue or loss of energy, feelings of worthlessness or excessive guilt, decreased concentration, and suicidal ideation. At least five of the symptoms must be present nearly every day for a period of 2 weeks or more to make the diagnosis of major depression. In addition, at least one of the symptoms must be depressed mood or loss of interest or pleasure. Antidepressant drugs are useful both in the treatment of acute episodes of major depression and in preventing recurrences of this disorder. Major depression with psychotic features generally responds best to a combination of an antidepressant and an antipsychotic drug, as discussed in chapter 1.

Bipolar Disorder, Depressed

Patients with bipolar disorder meet the criteria for major depression, but also have a history of one or more manic episodes. Although lithium and carbamazepine are the drugs of choice for preventing recurrences of mania or depression in bipolar patients, they are generally not as effective as the antidepressants in treating an acute depressive episode.

Dysthymia (or Depressive Neurosis)

Dysthymia is a chronic disorder of 2 or more years' duration with several of the features of major depression (e.g., disturbances in sleep and appetite; low energy or fatigue). However, dysthymia is less severe than major depression. It is best described as a chronic, mild depressive syndrome. The data supporting the use of antidepressants in this disorder are not as conclusive as those for major depression. However, a significant percentage of patients with dysthymia do respond to antidepressant treatment.

Atypical Depression

Although atypical depression is not listed in DSM-III-R as a distinct entity (it would be classified as Depressive Disorder Not Otherwise Specified), it is referred to in most texts and is therefore discussed here. Atypical depressions are characterized by significant anxiety, hypersomnia, increased appetite, fatigue, somatic complaints, phobias, obsessive symptoms, and sensitivity to rejection. They present as chronic conditions, generally without such features as self-reproach and suicidal ideation. These depressions have been reported to respond preferentially to the MAO inhibitors.

Panic Disorder, with or without Agoraphobia

Panic attacks are described in the DSM-III-R as "discrete periods of intense fear or discomfort." Patients report acute, almost-incapacitating anxiety that usually lasts for several minutes. In addition to the severe anxiety, these attacks are characterized by physical symptoms such as dizziness, palpitations, dyspnea, sweating, hot flashes, chest pain or discomfort, and nausea. Some patients report a fear of dying or going crazy. Panic disorder responds to treatment with MAO inhibitors, tricyclic antidepressants, and the benzodiazepines alprazolam and clonazepam. Among the tricyclic antidepressants, imipramine has been the most extensively studied and widely used. With the one exception of trazodone, all of the cyclic antidepressants that have been studied have been found to be effective in the prevention of panic attacks.

Enuresis

Enuresis, occurring mainly in children and adolescents, has been found to respond to tricyclic antidepressants. Imipramine in doses of 25 to 75 mg, given 1 hour before bedtime, has been most frequently used. However, higher doses may be required. Although it is generally effective and acts rapidly in this condition, there is no residual improvement when the drug is withdrawn. Thus, imipramine is primarily for temporary relief and should be combined with behavioral techniques when used in the treatment of enuresis.

Attention-Deficit Hyperactivity Disorder

Attention-deficit hyperactivity disorder (ADHD) was formerly called minimum brain dysfunction syndrome with hyperactivity. It is characterized by "developmentally inappropriate degrees of inattention, impulsiveness, and hyperactivity" according to DSM-III-R. The tricyclic antidepressants imipramine and desipramine have been found to be effective in the treatment of children with this disorder. As in the treatment of enuresis, response to the tricyclics occurs rapidly. However, tolerance to the beneficial effects of the tricyclics may develop after an initial effective response, and there is a high risk of relapse following withdrawal of the drugs. Thus, the CNS stimulants (e.g., methylphenidate, dextroamphetamine) remain the drugs of choice for ADHD at the present time.

Chronic Pain

Tricyclic antidepressants have been found to be effective in the treatment of a wide variety of chronic pain syndromes (e.g., headaches, fibrositis, chronic back pain, arthritis). Many patients are depressed secondary to their chronic pain. Some pain syndromes may represent a "depressive equivalent." However, the antidepressants have analgesic properties above and beyond their effect on depression. They are useful alone or in combination with other analgesics. Some clinicians prefer the more sedative tricyclics (e.g., amitriptyline, doxepin, trimipramine) for use in the treatment of chronic pain syndromes, giving the entire dose 2 hours before bedtime to facilitate sleep. In general, lower doses than those required to treat depression are effective in the treatment of chronic pain. The onset of action also occurs earlier than the antidepressant effect of these drugs. As a general rule, the starting dose of an antidepressant in the treatment of chronic pain should be about 25 mg of amitriptyline or the equivalent dose of another drug. The dose can then be gradually titrated upward to achieve maximum therapeutic benefit. The newer antidepressant fluoxetine also appears to be promising in the treatment of chronic pain.

Bulimia Nervosa

Patients with bulimia nervosa have recurrent episodes of binge eating, in which they consume a large amount of food in a short period of time. During the eating binges, they experience a lack of control over their eating behavior. Bulimic patients also engage in self-induced vomiting, the use of laxatives, strict dieting, or vigorous exercise in an attempt to prevent weight gain. According to DSM-III-R, there must be at least two binge eating episodes a week for at least 3 months and a "persistent overconcern with body shape and weight" in order to make the diagnosis of bulimia nervosa. Several tricyclic antidepressants and the MAO inhibitors phenelzine and tranylcypromine have been shown to be effective in controlling the binge eating of bulimic patients. Tricyclic antidepressants that are less likely to stimulate appetite and weight gain (e.g., desipramine) are the recommended drugs in this class for the treatment of bulimia. Experience with fluoxetine in the treatment of bulimic patients has also been favorable.

Obsessive Compulsive Disorder

OCD is characterized by recurrent obsessions (thoughts) and/or compulsions (acts) that are severe enough to cause marked distress or significantly interfere with an individual's occupational or social functioning. The obsessions or compulsions are time-consuming in that they take more than an hour a day. The treatment of choice for this disorder is one of the newer antidepressants, clomipramine (Anafranil) or fluoxetine (Prozac). Although more controlled studies have documented the effectiveness of clomipramine, clinical experience with fluoxetine has also been positive. Pharmacotherapy is effective in controlling both the obsessions and the compulsions of this disorder. Maximal therapeutic benefit may take up to 3 months of drug treatment. Patients generally report a gradual decrease in the intensity of their obsessions and compulsions. Behavioral modification techniques are also helpful in this disorder, especially for those patients with compulsions.

Narcolepsy

Narcolepsy, a neurologic disorder, is characterized by irresistible sleep attacks and by cataplexy, a sudden loss of muscular tone associated with emotional arousal. Both the tricyclic antidepressants and MAO inhibitors are effective in treating cataplexy. Protriptyline, the tricyclic antidepressant with stimulating properties, has become the drug of choice for the treatment of cataplexy. CNS stimulants (e.g., methylphenidate, dextroamphetamine) are used to treat the sleep attacks.

Sleep Apnea

There are three types of sleep apnea (obstructive, central, and mixed). All three are characterized by the cessation of breathing during sleep. Patients may actually stop breathing hundreds of times each night as they enter the deeper stages of sleep. Their sleep then lightens and breathing resumes. The patient is unaware of the apneic episodes, but complains of daytime fatigue and sleepiness. Obstructive sleep apnea is the most common form of the disorder and is secondary to a narrowing of the airways in the pharynx and hypopharynx such that air flow is obstructed. The tricyclic antidepressants protriptyline and imipramine (in conventional doses) have been effective in some cases of obstructive sleep apnea.

Phobic Disorders

Agoraphobia is characterized by a fear of being in places or situations from which escape might be difficult or embarrassing or in which help might not be readily available (DSM-III-R). Patients may restrict their activities to the point that they become housebound. Most patients with agoraphobia experience panic attacks, but this disorder may occur without panic attacks or with only limited symptom attacks. Agoraphobia has been found to be responsive to tricyclic antidepressants, MAO inhibitors, and alprazolam. Among the antidepressants, imipramine and phenelzine have been the most extensively studied and commonly used drugs in the treatment of this disorder. Response to treatment may occur more rapidly than that seen with depression.

Patients with social phobia have a persistent fear of situations in which they are exposed to possible scrutiny by others. They fear that they may do something or say something that will be humiliating or embarrassing. Some patients fear most social situations (global social phobia) while other patients may fear only certain situations (discrete or circumscribed social phobia). The fear of public speaking is a common discrete social phobia. MAO inhibitors, primarily phenelzine, have been found to be effective in the treatment of global social phobia. Discrete social phobias may respond preferentially to beta-blockers such as propranolol (Inderal). Experience with fluoxetine in the treatment of global social phobia has also been promising.

Peptic Ulcer Disease

Because of their H_2 histamine receptor blocking activity, the tricyclic antidepressants doxepin, amitriptyline, and trimipramine have been found to be effective in the treatment of peptic ulcer. The histamine H_2 receptor mediates the secretion of gastric acid. Although this indication is still in the investigational stage (tricyclic antidepressants are not the primary drugs used in the treatment of peptic ulcer), clinical trials with tricyclics have been promising.

GUIDELINES FOR CLINICAL USE

Treatment of Depression

Tricyclic and Tetracyclic Antidepressants

With the possible exception of doxepin, all of the tricyclics and tetracyclics appear to be about equal in overall efficacy. Doxepin may be less potent because it is a weaker inhibitor of neurotransmitter reuptake. Although nortriptyline and protriptyline are more potent on a milligram-per-milligram basis than the other drugs in this class, they are not more efficacious when the latter drugs are used in equivalent doses. All of the tricyclics and tetracyclics have a delay in their onset of action, taking an average of 2 to 4 weeks to exert their antidepressant effect. Claims that amoxapine has a more rapid onset of action require further substantiation. The two most common errors in prescribing these drugs are using too low a dose and not administering them for a long enough period of time to be effective. Although the selection of an appropriate drug based on laboratory measures (e.g., urinary MHPG [3-methoxy

4-hydroxyphenylglycol] excretion) holds promise, the choice of a tricyclic or tetracyclic for any given patient must be made on clinical grounds. As with the antipsychotics, a personal or family drug-response history may be useful in the selection of a drug. The clinician must also take into account the degree of sedative, anticholinergic, and α-adrenergic blocking properties of each of the tricyclic or tetracyclic antidepressants. For example, amitriptyline would be an appropriate choice for a depressed patient with anxiety and insomnia because of its strong sedative properties. Desipramine might be the drug of choice for a patient in whom anticholinergic side effects could be troublesome (e.g., a patient with prostatic hypertrophy or glaucoma). For a depressed patient with lethargy, psychomotor retardation, or hypersomnia, protriptyline could be used. For patients in whom orthostatic hypotension could prove troublesome (e.g., the elderly, those with cardiovascular problems), nortriptyline or desipramine would be an appropriate choice.

Once a tricyclic or tetracyclic has been selected for a patient, the following general guidelines apply to its clinical use. Although imipramine is used in the following sections, equivalent doses of other drugs could be substituted.

1. Using imipramine as an example, treatment could be started with 25 mg tid or 50 mg hs. If this regimen is well tolerated, the dose could then be increased by 25 to 50 mg every 3 to 4 days until a dose of 150 mg/d is reached. Although some patients (particularly less-depressed outpatients) may respond to a lower dose, most clinicians use 150 mg/d as an arbitrary end point. However, for severely depressed inpatients, the dose could be increased more rapidly and a higher end point (e.g., 200 to 250 mg) could be used.

2. Initially the dose could be given in a divided regimen. Along with gradual increases in dose, this tends to minimize side effects and allows for better titration of the drug. However, if the patient tolerates the medication well, it could be shifted to a single hs dose. This may help provide sedation for sleep, avoid excessive daytime sedation, and decrease the intensity of anticholinergic side effects and postural hypotension during the day. The main problem with a single large hs dose is the development of postural (orthostatic) hypotension and fainting if the patient gets up at night. However, if the dose is increased gradually (as noted previously), this is often not a problem. Instructing the patient to change positions (e.g., lying to standing) gradually often helps avoid symptoms secondary to postural hypotension. Patients with pretreatment postural hypotension are at greater risk for the development of further orthostatic decreases in blood pressure with tricyclic and tetracyclic drugs. Some patients experience nightmares with single large bedtime doses and do better with a divided dose regimen. If a single hs dose is not feasible, one third of the dose could be given during the day with two thirds given at bedtime.

3. This regimen would need to be modified for elderly patients and those with cardiovascular problems. The starting dose should be less and should be increased on a more gradual basis, and the initial end point should be between 50 mg and 100 mg/d. A divided dose regimen is also recommended. In general, starting and maintenance doses for the elderly should be approximately one third to one half of those for younger adults.

4. After a dose of 150 mg/d has been reached, the patient should be left on that dose for approximately 2 weeks. At that time response to treatment should be evaluated. The earliest signs of improvement are often changes in

appetite and sleep pattern. Although the full antidepressant effect of the tricyclics is generally not apparent for 2 to 4 weeks, patients may report improvement in sleep, appetite, and level of anxiety after only a few days. This is especially true of the more sedating tricyclics such as amitriptyline or doxepin. Other signs of improvement to look for at this time are an increase in general activity level and a renewal of social interests. Some change in mood should also be apparent. If improvement is satisfactory, the patient should be left on the 150 mg/d dosage.

5. If no definite signs of improvement are apparent (or if improvement is not optimal) after 2 weeks, and presuming the drug is well tolerated, the dose should be gradually increased by 25 to 50 mg every 3 to 4 days to a maximum of 300 mg/d. In general, the dose can be increased (up to 300 mg/d), until improvement is noted or troublesome side effects intervene. Patients often develop tolerance to the sedative side effects of tricyclics. Anticholinergic effects and postural hypotension may prove more troublesome. Some clinicians have found bethanechol (Urecholine) in doses up to 100 mg/d useful in the management of anticholinergic side effects.

6. For nortriptyline, imipramine, and desipramine, measuring plasma levels may be helpful in establishing an effective treatment dose. Only for these three tricyclics are there good data correlating plasma level with clinical response. Therapeutic plasma levels for these drugs are as follows:

- nortriptyline: 50 to 150 ng/mL
- imipramine (+Desipramine): 200 to 300 ng/mL
- desipramine: 100 to 250 ng/mL

Plasma levels are especially helpful in patients who do not respond to routine doses, in elderly or medically ill patients, and in those experiencing troublesome side effects. It is important to remember that there may be as much as a tenfold (or more) difference in plasma levels among patients receiving the same dose of a tricyclic. This fact underscores the need to individualize the treatment dose with tricyclics. Table 2.4 lists normative dose ranges for antidepressants, but some patients will fall outside these ranges.

7. After maximal dosage has been reached, the patient should be left on that regimen for approximately 4 to 6 weeks. This represents an adequate clinical trial. If improvement is not optimal by that time, the patient should be considered refractory to the drug and another treatment should be instituted.

8. After a patient has responded optimally to a tricyclic or tetracyclic antidepressant, the issue of maintenance treatment arises. Recent studies have demonstrated the need for longer-term maintenance treatment to prevent relapse. It is recommended that the patient recovering from an initial episode of depression be left on the dose that he or she has responded to for approximately 3 to 4 months. This ensures that maximal benefit will be obtained from the drug and decreases the risk of relapse. After this time period the dose may be gradually tapered by 25 mg every 1 or 2 weeks (or even more slowly) until an effective maintenance level is reached. As a general guideline, an adequate maintenance dose can be thought of as being approximately one half the therapeutic dose. However, there may be considerable variation from patient to patient and some patients may require maintenance treatment with the full therapeutic dose. If a patient shows signs of relapse as the dose is being de-

creased, the last previously effective dose should be reinstituted. Often, the earliest signs of relapse are insomnia and irritability.

9. Maintenance treatment should be continued until such time as the patient has been symptom-free for 6 to 12 months. Patients with recurrent episodes of depression and/or a positive family history of depression require longer maintenance treatment than patients with no prior history of depressive illness. After several months of maintenance therapy, the drug should be gradually discontinued. During this phase of treatment, the dose could be decreased by 25 mg/wk until it is completely discontinued. Again, should there be any signs of relapse, the last previously effective dose should be reinstituted. Tricyclic and tetracyclic drugs should never be discontinued abruptly. A gradual tapering of the dose allows for early detection of any signs of relapse and permits the physician to promptly reinstitute an effective therapeutic dose. Abrupt discontinuation of these drugs has also been associated with symptoms of cholinergic rebound. Patients may experience nausea, vomiting, headache, sweating, and general malaise.

10. Some patients with severe depressions may require prolonged maintenance therapy, while those with frequent recurrent bouts of depression or chronic depression may need maintenance treatment indefinitely. For these patients, the lowest possible dose that will prevent a recurrence of symptoms should be used. Long-term treatment with tricyclics or tetracyclics has not been associated with any major side effects. This is in contrast to long-term treatment with antipsychotic drugs, which may cause tardive dyskinesia. However, long-term treatment with amoxapine does pose a risk for the development of tardive dyskinesia because of its dopamine receptor blocking effects.

11. Unlike the antipsychotic drugs, which have a wide margin of safety, the tricyclic and tetracyclic antidepressants can be fatal if an overdose is taken. Approximately ten times the therapeutic dose can be a lethal dose. Since many depressed patients are suicide-prone, it is a good idea not to prescribe more than a week's supply of medication at a time. In this regard it is important to keep in mind that nortriptyline and protriptyline are more potent than the other drugs in this class and that a lesser amount of these drugs could be fatal if taken in overdose. Amoxapine, on the other hand, is the least potent drug of this class on a milligram-per-milligram basis.

12. If a patient is refractory to any given tricyclic or tetracyclic, several treatment options are available to the clinician. Switching to another tricyclic is one option (e.g., if a patient is refractory to a tertiary amine tricyclic, he or she could be tried on a secondary amine tricyclic). However, it may prove more fruitful to try one of the atypical antidepressants or a MAO inhibitor. Another option would be to add lithium to the tricyclic or tetracyclic drug. Lithium augmentation of tricyclics and tetracyclics and MAO inhibitors has been helpful to many treatment-resistant patients. Many clinicians prefer to try this option first, as the response to lithium augmentation may be apparent within 1 week. It is thought that lithium potentiates serotonergic activity and thus enhances the response to antidepressant drugs. When lithium is used in this fashion, doses in the range of 300 mg tid are generally employed. Yet another option is to add triiodothyronine (T_3) (Cytomel) to the antidepressant drug. Doses in the range of 25 to 50 mcq/d of T_3 have been helpful to some treatment-refractory patients. However, augmentation with T_3 is not felt to be as effective

as lithium augmentation. Patients who respond to T_3 may have a subtle form of thyroid dysfunction.

13. If a patient has been refractory to two or three different antidepressants and the previously recommended augmentation techniques, then electroconvulsive therapy (ECT) should be considered. ECT has been shown to be an effective treatment for depression (generally more effective than the antidepressant drugs) and is indicated in the following situations:

- in depressed patients who are refractory to the antidepressant drugs
- in severely depressed patients who are acutely suicidal. ECT acts more rapidly than the antidepressant drugs, which have a delay in their onset of action
- in depressed patients with medical contraindications to antidepressant drugs (e.g., cardiac conduction abnormalities)
- in patients with a past history of response to ECT

MAO Inhibitors

Much of what has been said in guidelines for the use of tricyclic and tetracyclic antidepressants also applies to the MAO inhibitors. However, there are some differences.

The usual starting dose for phenelzine is 15 mg bid or 15 mg tid. If this dose is well tolerated by the patient, it can then be increased by 15 mg increments to 60 mg/d by the end of the first week to 10 days of treatment. This is often an effective therapeutic dose, and the patient should be left on this regimen for approximately 2 to 3 weeks. If no improvement is seen at the end of this time, and there are no adverse effects, the dose may be increased at a rate of 15 mg/wk up to a maximum daily dose of 90 mg/d. This is generally regarded as the upper dose limit for phenelzine. Four weeks at 90 mg/d represents an adequate clinical trial, and if no improvement is seen at the end of this time, the drug should be discontinued. However, it may take 6 weeks for optimal improvement to be seen with phenelzine. The usual effective daily dose range for phenelzine is 45 to 90 mg/d. Some clinicians recommend aiming for 1 mg/kg of body weight to achieve a therapeutic dose for phenelzine. As with the tricyclics and tetracyclics, after the patient has responded optimally to a given dose of phenelzine, he or she should be left on that dose for approximately 3 to 4 months to avoid relapse. After that time the dosage may be gradually decreased to a maintenance level. However, maintenance regimens for MAO inhibitors have not been as well established as they have for tricyclic antidepressants. Thus some clinicians recommend leaving the patient on the full therapeutic dose for 6 to 12 months after he or she has been symptom-free and then gradually discontinuing the drug.

Tranylcypromine is more potent than phenelzine on a milligram-per-milligram basis, and the starting and peak doses are lower. The starting dose for tranylcypromine is 10 mg bid. If there is no response after 1 to 2 weeks and the drug is well-tolerated, it can be increased by 10 mg/wk up to a maximal daily dose of 50 mg/d (some clinicians recommend going as high as 60 mg/d for severely depressed, refractory patients). Thirty mg/d of tranylcypromine is often an effective dose, and 10 to 14 days on this dose represents an adequate therapeutic trial for many patients. For those who do not respond, the dose can be cautiously increased as noted previously. Tranylcypromine has a quicker onset of action than phenelzine and the tricyclic antidepressants. This may be due to its amphetamine-like stimulating effects. The starting and therapeutic doses for isocarboxazid are similar to those for tranylcypromine. An initial dose of 10 mg bid could be employed, with most patients requiring no more than 30 mg/d. Some patients have required up to 50 mg/d, and this is the upper dose limit for isocarboxazid. As noted before, this drug is less commonly prescribed than phenelzine and tranylcypromine.

Unlike the tricyclics, excessive sedation and anticholinergic effects are not common problems with MAO inhibitors. However, orthostatic hypotension and excessive CNS stimulation may be troublesome. As noted before, hypertensive crises may occur if patients do not adhere to a tyramine-free diet. Because of the long duration of enzyme inhibition, MAO inhibitors can be given on a once-a-day basis after a patient has been stabilized on divided daily doses. This is best accomplished by gradually shifting the doses to a single daily dose in the morning. Single daily bedtime doses may cause insomnia because of excessive stimulation.

Like the tricyclics, MAO inhibitors have a narrow margin of safety and can be fatal if an overdose is taken. Approximately ten times the therapeutic dose of phenelzine can be a lethal dose. For tranylcypromine and isocarboxazid the margin of safety is even less. The same precautions necessary in prescribing tricyclic antidepressants apply to the MAO inhibitors. A controversial topic has been the combined use of a tricyclic antidepressant and a MAO inhibitor. Theoretically, this combination would appear to be rational as the two classes of drugs exert their antidepressant effects by different mechanisms. However, drug company manufacturers and most textbooks recommend a 10- to 14-day "washout period" of one drug before starting the other. This is in response to reports of hyperpyrexia, hypertensive crises, convulsions, and even death in patients who were on a combination of a tricyclic and a MAO inhibitor. However, there have been several reports in the literature from this country and Europe that the combination is both safe and effective and that it produces no more side effects than either drug alone. Some authors recommend combined treatment with a tricyclic and a MAO inhibitor for those patients who are refractory to usual doses of either drug alone. The combination has been reported to be effective in these cases. It may also be useful for patients who respond only to very high doses of tricyclics and who are bothered by their associated side effects. When using this combination, it is recommended that the tricyclic antidepressant be started first and that the MAO inhibitor then be added slowly. Alternatively, both drugs can be cautiously started concurrently. A tricyclic antidepressant should never be added to a MAO inhibitor. The combination of amitriptyline and phenelzine seems to be the safest and is most commonly used. The final dose of both is generally lower than when either drug is used alone, 150 mg of amitriptyline and 30 mg of phenelzine often being an effective regimen. Doxepin and trimipramine have also been used in combination with phenelzine. Desipramine and imipramine should *not* be used. Also, tranylcypromine is not recommended for use in combination with a tricyclic antidepressant.

It should be noted that controlled studies are needed to document the efficacy and safety of this combination before it can be recommended for routine clinical use. Nevertheless, it may be justified for those patients refractory to standard treatment regimens (including ECT). If the combination is to be employed, it should be done so cautiously and only by an experienced clinician. The informed consent of the patient and/or his family should be obtained.

Notwithstanding the preceding discussion on combination tricyclic-MAO inhibitor treatment, certain precautions need to be taken when making a transition between other antidepressants and MAO inhibitors to avoid potentially serious drug interactions.

1. When switching from a MAO inhibitor to a tricyclic antidepressant, the patient should be off the MAO inhibitor for 14 days before initiating treatment with the tricyclic, because it takes the body about 10 to 14 days to regenerate MAO. For this reason patients should also be advised to follow their dietary restrictions for 14 days after discontinuing a MAO inhibitor.

2. When switching from a tricyclic antidepressant to a MAO inhibitor, the patient should be off the tricyclic for 7 days before initiating treatment with the MAO inhibitor.

3. When switching from a MAO inhibitor to one of the atypical antidepressants (bupropion, fluoxetine, or trazodone), a 14-day "washout period" (as for the tricyclics) is recommended before initiating treatment with one of the atypical antidepressants.

4. When switching from fluoxetine to a MAO inhibitor, the patient should be off fluoxetine for 5 weeks before initiating treatment with the MAO inhibitor, because of the very long half-life of fluoxetine and its active metabolite.

5. When switching from bupropion or trazodone to a MAO inhibitor, a "washout period" of 7 days before initiating treatment with the MAO inhibitor should be sufficient.

6. Care must also be taken when switching from one MAO inhibitor to another, especially when switching from phenelzine to tranylcypromine. After discontinuing treatment with one MAO inhibitor, a 14-day drug-free period is recommended before initiating treatment with another MAO inhibitor.

Atypical Antidepressants

The guidelines for use of the atypical antidepressants are similar to those for the tricyclics. The specific features of bupropion, fluoxetine, and trazodone have been discussed previously in individual sections on each drug.

In general, starting doses for the atypical antidepressants should be low and gradually increased into the therapeutic range. The manufacturer recommends starting bupropion at 100 mg bid, but a lower starting dose of 100 to 150 mg/d may be preferable. The dose can then be gradually increased until a positive therapeutic response is seen. The total daily dose of bupropion should not exceed 450 mg, and no more than 150 mg should be given as a single dose to reduce the risk of seizures with this drug. The recommended starting dose for fluoxetine is 20 mg/d, given in the morning to minimize its tendency to produce insomnia. Because of the long half-life of fluoxetine, dose increases of this drug should be more gradual (e.g., every 2 to 3 weeks) than with other antidepressants. The maximum recommended dose of fluoxetine is 80 mg/d. Doses above 20 mg/d should be given in a divided regimen. Trazodone can be started at 50 to 100 mg/d. As this drug is highly sedating, a bedtime dose is often better tolerated. The dose can then be gradually increased up to a maximal daily dose of 400 mg/d for outpatients and 600 mg/d for inpatients.

Higher doses should be given in a divided regimen. Although maintenance doses for the newer drugs (bupropion and fluoxetine) have not been established, it is reasonable to assume that (as with the tricyclics) lower doses may be sufficient for maintenance treatment. Thus, after the patient has been stabilized for 3 to 4 months, the dose can be gradually decreased to the lowest effective level.

Approximate daily dose ranges for all the antidepressants are listed in Table 2.4.

SIDE EFFECTS

Tricyclic and Tetracyclic Antidepressants

Anticholinergic Effects
Minor side effects include dry mouth, constipation, excessive sweating, tachycardia, pupillary dilatation, and blurred vision. More severe side effects include urinary hesitancy and retention, paralytic ileus, exacerbation of narrow-angle glaucoma, and a toxic confusional state (delirium). Tricyclics should be prescribed with caution in patients with glaucoma or prostatic hypertrophy. Dry mouth, xerostomia, can result in stomatitis or dental caries. Advising the patient to increase his or her fluid intake and to chew sugarless gum is usually helpful in controlling this side effect. An increased fluid intake and a diet high in fiber is often sufficient in controlling constipation. Bethanechol may be helpful in counteracting anticholinergic effects, especially urinary hesitancy. Doses in the range of 10 to 25 mg tid or qid are generally used. The elderly are at greater risk for developing an anticholinergic delirium, which may also be seen with overdoses of tricyclics along with other signs of excess anticholinergic activity. Treatment is with physostigmine (Antilirium) 1 to 2 mg intramuscularly (IM) or *slowly* intravenously (IV). If given IV, physostigmine should be given at a rate of no more than 1 mg/min. The dose may need to be repeated at 30 to 45 minute intervals until symptoms clear permanently. Tolerance often develops to the milder anticholinergic side effects.

Cardiovascular Effects
Postural hypotension, tachycardia, and palpitations are the most common side effects. The tricyclics also have a quinidine-like action and can produce changes in cardiac conduction. The ECG may show prolongation of the PR interval, prolongation of the QT interval, depression of the ST segment, flattening of the T wave, and more rarely, bundle branch block. Cardiac arrhythmias (both supraventricular and ventricular) may occur, particularly following an overdose. In general, arrhythmias are rare in patients with healthy hearts when therapeutic doses of tricyclics are employed. Patients with a history of cardiac disease are at a greater risk for the development of arrhythmias, and the tricyclics must be used with caution in this population. Direct suppression of the myocardium and the precipitation of congestive heart failure have also been reported. Tricyclics are not recommended during the acute recovery phase following a myocardial infarction. Postural (orthostatic) hypotension is a far more common and potentially limiting complication of tricyclic treatment. The elderly and medically debilitated patients are at greater risk for its develop-

ment. It can often be minimized by gradual dose increases and instructing the patient to change positions slowly. Tolerance to this side effect often occurs after several weeks of treatment, and it may also respond to a reduction in dose. Nortriptyline is the tricyclic antidepressant least likely to produce postural hypotension.

Antihistaminic Effects

Excessive sedation may occur with the tricyclics, especially those with significant antihistaminic effects (doxepin, trimipramine, and amitriptyline). This side effect can be managed clinically by giving the entire dose, or a large part of it, at bedtime. This generally ensures a good night's sleep and minimizes daytime sedation.

Weight gain is another side effect felt to be related to the antihistaminic effect of the tricyclics. It can be quite pronounced in some patients, who often report a craving for carbohydrates. If it becomes problematic, switching the patient to a less antihistaminic tricyclic or to one of the atypical antidepressants (bupropion, fluoxetine, or trazodone) may be helpful. Bupropion and trazodone have not been associated with weight gain, and fluoxetine may actually cause weight loss.

CNS Effects

Tricyclics can produce a fine tremor because of their adrenergic effects. If this side effect is problematic, it can be treated with a beta-blocker such as propranolol.

Some patients will report restlessness, jitteriness, insomnia, or agitation secondary to treatment with tricyclics. Should this occur, switching to a more sedative tricyclic may prove helpful. Another option would be to add a benzodiazepine to the tricyclic. The combination drug Limbitrol (amitriptyline and chlordiazepoxide) may be useful for those patients who experience restlessness or jitteriness on a tricyclic alone. For patients who experience more severe agitation on a tricyclic, the combination of amitriptyline and perphenazine may be helpful. However, the clinician must weigh the risk of the possibility of tardive dyskinesia if perphenazine is employed.

The tricyclics may precipitate a hypomanic or manic episode in predisposed patients. Patients with a previous history of bipolar disorder or hypomania or those with a family history of bipolar disorder are at greater risk for the development of a drug-induced manic episode. Tricyclics may also precipitate or exacerbate a psychotic episode in a patient with a history of schizophrenia. If either of these reactions occurs, the tricyclic should be withdrawn. The combination of amitriptyline and perphenazine may be useful for depressed patients with a history of schizophrenia.

Like the antipsychotic drugs, the tricyclics lower the convulsive threshold and may cause seizures in susceptible patients. This is an uncommon side effect. However, doses of anticonvulsants may need to be adjusted in patients with epilepsy. Maprotiline appears to be at a higher risk for the induction of seizures than the other drugs in this class and is contraindicated in patients with a previous history of seizure disorder. Epileptics can be cautiously treated with the other tricyclics.

Some patients report nightmares after taking their entire dose of tricyclic at bedtime. This can be managed clinically by administering the drug in divided daily doses. Speech blocking may be seen, particularly with the more sedating and anticholinergic tricyclics.

Other Side Effects
At times, other side effects may occur with the use of tricyclic and tetracyclic antidepressants. Skin rashes appear to be more frequent with maprotiline. They represent an allergic reaction and occur early in the course of treatment. Sexual dysfunction is not uncommonly reported by patients taking tricyclics. Impotence and retarded ejaculation may be seen. These often respond to switching to a less-anticholinergic antidepressant. Both increased and decreased libido have been reported. An increase in libido may be expected as the patient's depression improves. Edema and myoclonus are infrequent side effects of tricyclics; cholestatic jaundice, purpura, and agranulocytosis, are rare side effects of tricyclics.

MAO Inhibitors

Orthostatic (Postural) Hypotension
Hypotension is the most common side effect associated with MAO inhibitors. It may present with symptoms of dizziness, lightheadedness, and occasionally fainting spells. Phenelzine is more hypotensive than tranylcypromine and isocarboxazid. Postural hypotension can be managed by using the lowest possible dose of medication in a divided-dose regimen. The patient should be instructed to change positions (from lying or sitting to standing) slowly. If these measures do not effectively control postural hypotension, increasing the patient's salt intake may be helpful. This should be done only in patients who can safely tolerate an increased sodium intake. Maintaining adequate hydration and the use of support stockings may also be helpful. Some clinicians recommend the use of fludrocortisone (Florinef), a salt-retaining steroid, for patients who do not respond to other measures. Total daily doses up to 0.6 to 0.8 mg have been employed. However, fludrocortisone carries the risks of hypokalemia, congestive heart failure, and hypertension. Thus it should be used cautiously and only in carefully selected patients.

CNS Effects
Overstimulation may occur as a result of the stimulating properties of MAO inhibitors. Clinically, patients may complain of agitation, restlessness, irritability, and insomnia. Phenelzine is the least stimulating MAO inhibitor and may produce sedation in some patients. Giving the majority of the dose in the morning may help alleviate insomnia. Daytime overstimulation may be helped by a reduction in dose. Patients should be instructed to avoid caffeinated beverages.

Like the tricyclics, the MAO inhibitors may precipitate manic or psychotic episodes in susceptible individuals. Hypertensive crises may occur in patients taking MAO inhibitors who ingest foods containing tyramine or medications containing sympathomimetic agents. These reactions are more commonly seen with tranylcypromine than with phenelzine. The overall incidence of these reactions is low, but they can be potentially fatal. Thus, strict adherence to the dietary restrictions listed in Table 2.5 must be maintained. As a general rule, patients should not take any new medication without consulting their physician. An acute hypertensive crisis presents with an intense, throbbing headache, flushing, sweating, nausea, and vomiting. Patients may also have a stiff neck and palpitations associated with the sudden and dramatic rise in blood pressure. Rare cases have resulted in intracranial bleeding and fatality. Patients should be instructed to seek prompt medical attention (i.e., go to a local emergency room) if these symptoms occur. The treatment of choice is phentolamine (Regitine) given slowly IV in a dose of 5 mg. Phentolamine is a short-acting α-adrenergic blocking drug. Some clinicians recommend that patients take 50 to 100 mg of chlorpromazine if they do not have immediate access to medical care. Chlorpromazine's alpha-blocking properties may prove useful, but could result in an uncontrolled hypotensive reaction. A more reasonable alternative may be the use of sublingual nifedipine in a dose of 10 mg. Nifedipine is a calcium channel blocker that has recently been found to be effective in controlling these hypertensive reactions without causing unwanted hypotension.

Hepatotoxicity

Hepatotoxicity is a rare side effect of MAO inhibitors. However, when it does occur, it is more serious than the cholestatic jaundice associated with the antipsychotic drugs and tricyclics. Parenchymal destruction of the liver can occur. The hydrazine MAO inhibitors carry a greater risk of hepatotoxicity, especially isocarboxazid. Tranylcypromine appears to be relatively safe in this regard.

Sexual Dysfunction

Decreased libido, impaired sexual arousal, impotence, ejaculatory disturbances, and anorgasmia have all been reported with MAO inhibitors. Reducing the dose may be helpful in alleviating sexual dysfunction. Some patients have found cyproheptadine (Periactin) in doses of 2 to 8 mg/d helpful in counteracting anorgasmia. Cyproheptadine is an antihistamine with potent antiserotonergic activity.

Weight Gain

As with the tricyclic antidepressants, some patients taking MAO inhibitors report an increased appetite and craving for carbohydrates with a resultant gain in weight.

Paresthesias and Muscle Pains

Paresthesias and muscle pains appear to be related to the MAO inhibitors interfering with pyridoxine (vitamin B_6) metabolism. Hydrazine drugs such as phenelzine and isocarboxazid can produce a pyridoxine deficiency. Paresthesias and muscle pains often respond to supplemental pyridoxine given in doses of approximately 100 mg/d.

Autonomic Side Effects
  Although MAO inhibitors do not block acetylcholine receptors, patients may develop dry mouth, constipation, and urinary hesitancy. These side effects may be secondary to an increase in noradrenergic activity. They may be helped by a reduction in dose to the lowest effective level.

Occasional Side Effects
  Occasional side effects of MAO inhibitors include skin rashes, edema, myoclonus, and leukopenia.

Rare Side Effects
  Rare side effects of MAO inhibitors include excessive flatus and a lupus-like syndrome. The latter has been reported only with the hydrazine derivatives.

USE IN PREGNANCY AND LACTATION

  Tricyclic antidepressants do not appear to cause fetal malformations. However, it is good practice to avoid the use of tricyclics during pregnancy whenever possible, especially during the first trimester. As with the antipsychotic drugs, whether or not to use a tricyclic during pregnancy requires good clinical judgment on the part of the physician and the informed consent of the patient. If a tricyclic must be used during the first trimester of pregnancy, it is preferable to choose one of the older, more-established agents. Drugs such as amitriptyline, desipramine, and imipramine have longer safety records than the newer agents. If antidepressant treatment is initiated in the last trimester of pregnancy, the use of imipramine or desipramine is preferable, as these drugs would have less in the way of anticholinergic and sedative effects on the newborn.
  MAO inhibitors have been found to cause fetal malformations in animal studies. Although there are no data regarding their teratogenic potential in humans, these drugs should be avoided during pregnancy. The tricyclic antidepressants offer a safer alternative should antidepressant treatment be necessary. The MAO inhibitors would also be likely to adversely affect the fetus's developing enzyme systems.
  The atypical antidepressants and the newer tricyclic and tetracyclic drugs do not have the long-established safety records of the drugs previously mentioned. Thus, they are not recommended as the drugs of choice for use during pregnancy.
  Tricyclic antidepressants are excreted in breast milk in variable concentrations. It is therefore advisable that mothers on antidepressants avoid breastfeeding their infants.

USE IN THE ELDERLY

  The tricyclic and tetracyclic antidepressants have several side effects that can be particularly troublesome for elderly patients. Excessive sedation may cause increased confusion and disorientation, as may the anticholinergic effects of these drugs. Anticholinergic effects are also responsible for urinary hesitancy and retention seen in elderly males with prostate problems. Postural hypotension may result in falls and subsequent fractures. The effect of tricyclics on cardiac conduction increases the risk of developing an arrhythmia in those patients with preexisting cardiac disease. Thus, those tricyclics with fewer sedative, anticholinergic, and cardiovascular side effects are recommended for use in the elderly. Desipramine, which is low in anticholinergic activity and sedation, is one of the preferred drugs for use in the elderly. Nortriptyline, which appears to be least likely to cause postural hypotension (and is also relatively low in its sedative and anticholinergic effects), is another good choice. Both of these drugs can also be monitored by serum levels to provide for better titration of dose. In general, tricyclics should be given in low, divided doses to elderly patients to minimize the impact of any adverse effects. Any dose increases should be very gradual. In general, starting and maintenance doses for the elderly should be approximately one third to one half of those for younger adults. However, there is considerable variation among patients, and serum levels are often useful in aiding the physician in determining the correct dose.

The MAO inhibitors have minimal anticholinergic effects, often do not cause sedation, and have no effect on cardiac conduction. However, they do cause significant postural hypotension, which poses a risk for the elderly. The elderly patient is also at greater risk to develop a cerebrovascular accident should a hypertensive crisis occur while taking a MAO inhibitor. Nevertheless, cautious use of a MAO inhibitor may be beneficial for carefully selected geriatric patients.

The atypical antidepressants have not been studied as extensively in the treatment of elderly patients. However, bupropion and fluoxetine have favorable side-effect profiles and appear to be good choices for the treatment of this age group. Both drugs produce little in the way of excessive sedation, anticholinergic, and cardiovascular side effects.

For some elderly depressed patients, especially those with concurrent medical illnesses, treatment with the psychostimulants (dextroamphetamine or methylphenidate) may be helpful. Although these drugs should be thought of as CNS stimulants rather than antidepressants, they can produce a positive short-term antidepressant effect in some patients. Outside of excessive stimulation and perhaps tachycardia, they produce little in the way of adverse side effects. Patients who are unable to tolerate the conventional antidepressant drugs may benefit from treatment with the psychostimulants. Methylphenidate (Ritalin) is generally used in doses of 5 to 10 mg two or three times per day. The dose range for dextroamphetamine is 5 mg two or three times per day. Because of the risks of tolerance and abuse, these drugs should generally be used on a short-term basis.

DRUG INTERACTIONS

Tricyclic and Tetracyclic Antidepressants

1. The central sedative effects of the tricyclics and tetracyclics are additive when given with other drugs that have CNS-depressant properties (e.g., alcohol, sedative-hypnotics, antianxiety agents, antihistamines, and antipsychotics). Oversedation can occur particularly when amitriptyline, doxepin, or trimipramine is combined with any of the other drugs.

2. The anticholinergic properties of the tricyclics and tetracyclics will also be additive to those of other drugs with anticholinergic effects (e.g., antiparkinsonian drugs, antihistamines, phenothiazines, and belladonna alkaloids).

3. The cardiotoxic effects of the tricyclics and tetracyclics are additive with those of thioridazine. Thus, the combination of thioridazine and one of these agents should be avoided. To a lesser extent the same holds true for chlorpromazine, which should also not be used in combination with a tricyclic or tetracyclic drug.

4. The effects of the antiarrhythmic drugs, quinidine and procainamide, on the heart are potentiated by the tricyclics and tetracyclics. Patients on one of these drugs for whom a tricyclic is indicated need to have their dosage of quinidine or procainamide adjusted accordingly or be switched to another antiarrhythmic agent. Some studies have shown that imipramine can actually be substituted for quinidine because of the similarity of their actions.

5. Tricyclics and tetracyclics block the action of guanethidine (Ismelin) and clonidine (Catapres) and thus reverse the hypotensive effects of these drugs. The exception to this effect is doxepin in doses of 150 mg/d or less.

6. Barbiturates increase the metabolism of tricyclic and tetracyclic antidepressants through the induction of hepatic microsomal enzymes. Thus, they decrease the plasma levels of tricyclics. Chloral hydrate, carbamazepine (Tegretol), alcohol, and tobacco smoking have also been reported to decrease the plasma levels of tricyclics and tetracyclics via enzyme induction. On the other hand, the benzodiazepines do not alter the serum levels of tricyclics.

7. Several drugs retard the metabolism of tricyclic and tetracyclic antidepressants and thus increase their plasma levels. These drugs include the phenothiazines, butyrophenones, cimetidine (Tagamet), disulfiram (Antabuse), isoniazid, methylphenidate (Ritalin), dextroamphetamine, and oral contraceptives.

8. The strong anticholinergic effects of the tricyclics slow down gastrointestinal motility and may interfere with the absorption of other drugs. This has been reported for levodopa and phenylbutazone. Other drugs may be similarly affected.

9. The plasma half-life of Dicumarol has been reported to be prolonged by nortriptyline. Patients on anticoagulants and tricyclics should be closely observed for this possibly serious interaction (increased bleeding time).

10. The tricyclics can potentiate the hypertensive and arrhythmia-producing effects of sympathomimetic amines (e.g., epinephrine, norepinephrine, phenylephrine). These agents are used as decongestants in cold preparations and in dental anesthetic preparations.

11. Thyroid hormone may increase plasma levels of tricyclic and tetracyclic antidepressants.

12. Aspirin may potentiate the antidepressant effect of tricyclic and tetracyclic drugs by displacing them from plasma protein binding sites.

MAO Inhibitors

The MAO inhibitors potentiate many different drugs. Some of the drug interactions produce serious adverse effects and may be potentially life-threatening. The following are some of the more important drug interactions of the MAO inhibitors.

1. Alcohol, barbiturates, chloral hydrate, benzodiazepines, and general anesthetics are all potentiated by MAO inhibitors. Other CNS depressants potentiated by the MAO inhibitors include antihistamines, phenothiazines, and narcotic analgesics.

2. The combination of a MAO inhibitor and meperidine (Demerol) has been associated with hyperpyrexia, seizures, extreme excitement, and reactions simulating a narcotic overdose. Coma and death have been reported from this combination. The use of a narcotic analgesic should be avoided in patients taking MAO inhibitors.

3. Insulin and oral hypoglycemic agents are also potentiated by MAO inhibitors. Thus, patients on antidiabetic medication and a MAO inhibitor need to be followed closely for signs of hypoglycemia. They may require a decrease in the dose of insulin or oral hypoglycemic agent.

4. Other drugs potentiated by MAO inhibitors include amphetamines, anticholinergic antiparkinsonian agents, other anticholinergic drugs, hypotensive diuretics, and smooth-muscle relaxants.

5. Drugs that are used for indications other than depression may also have MAO-inhibiting activity. The combination of one of these drugs with phenelzine, tranylcypromine, or isocarboxazid could result in a toxic reaction characterized by hypertension, hyperpyrexia, CNS excitation, and seizures. Drugs in this category include:

- *pargyline (Eutonyl)*, a MAO inhibitor marketed as an antihypertensive agent
- *furazolidone (Furoxone)*, an antibiotic
- *procarbazine (Matulane)*, an antineoplastic agent used in the treatment of Hodgkin's disease
- *selegiline (Eldepryl; L-deprenyl)*, a MAO inhibitor used in the treatment of Parkinson's disease

6. Hypertensive crises have been reported when MAO inhibitors were used in combination with levodopa. However, carbidopa does not appear to produce this effect.

7. When MAO inhibitors have been used with reserpine and alpha-methyldopa, acute paradoxical hypertension and CNS excitation have been reported.

8. MAO inhibitors prolong the activity of succinylcholine, a muscle relaxant used in conjunction with ECT. MAO inhibitors should be discontinued 2 weeks before ECT is initiated. ECT itself can potentially cause hypertension if used concomitantly with a MAO inhibitor because of the increased release of catecholamines secondary to ECT.

9. MAO inhibitors should not be used in patients with suspected pheochromocytoma or carcinoid syndrome because of the risk of hypertensive reactions.

10. The combination of L-tryptophan and a MAO inhibitor may cause a serotonergic syndrome characterized by diaphoresis, hyperreflexia, myoclonus (muscle jerks), restlessness, nausea, and diarrhea.

11. The interaction between MAO inhibitors and tricyclic antidepressants has been discussed previously. This combination may not be as toxic as was once thought and may prove to be therapeutically useful in cases of refrac-

tory depression. However, proper precautions, as previously discussed, must be taken.

12. Foods containing tyramine and medications containing sympathomimetic agents must be avoided by patients taking MAO inhibitors to prevent the risk of developing a hypertensive crisis. Foods and drugs to be avoided are listed in Table 2.5.

13. The combination of buspirone (Buspar) and a MAO inhibitor may cause an elevation in blood pressure. This combination should be avoided.

14. The combination of cocaine and a MAO inhibitor has been reported to cause an elevation in blood pressure and a transient acute psychosis. Because cocaine is a popular drug of abuse, patients taking a MAO inhibitor should be warned about this potential interaction.

Atypical Antidepressants

Because the atypical antidepressants are relatively new, less is known about the potential drug interactions that might occur with them. Thus appropriate cautions should be taken when these drugs are used with other agents, particularly other CNS-acting drugs. Some potential drug interactions with these agents are noted here.

1. The combination of bupropion and a MAO inhibitor may result in a toxic reaction and thus should be avoided.

2. The combination of bupropion and L-dopa has been reported to cause a higher incidence of adverse reactions. This is most likely due to bupropion's inhibition of dopamine reuptake, which would potentiate the effect of L-dopa. If this combination is used, bupropion should be added cautiously to patients receiving L-dopa.

3. Bupropion must also be used cautiously with other drugs that lower the seizure threshold because of the increased risk of seizure induction with this antidepressant.

4. Bupropion may induce hepatic microsomal enzymes and thus could theoretically lower the blood levels of other coadministered drugs.

5. Drugs that induce hepatic microsomal enzymes (e.g., barbiturates, carbamazepine) would be expected to lower the plasma levels of bupropion, fluoxetine, and trazodone.

6. Drugs that inhibit or retard the hepatic metabolism of other drugs (e.g., cimetidine, phenothiazines, methylphenidate) would be expected to raise the plasma levels of bupropion, fluoxetine, and trazodone.

7. Fluoxetine should not be used in combination with MAO inhibitors because of the risk of severe toxic reactions. Appropriate precautions for switching from fluoxetine to a MAO inhibitor and vice-versa have been previously discussed.

8. The combination of L-tryptophan and fluoxetine has been reported to cause agitation, restlessness, and gastrointestinal distress. These symptoms are most likely due to excessive serotonergic activity.

9. Fluoxetine has been reported to increase the plasma levels of other antidepressants when given concomitantly with these drugs. Greater than two-fold increases in plasma levels of other antidepressants have been noted. Appropriate monitoring of patients on this combination is warranted.

10. When fluoxetine has been used in combination with lithium, both increased and decreased serum lithium levels have been reported. There have been reports of lithium toxicity on this combination, and close monitoring of serum lithium levels is warranted.

11. Fluoxetine may prolong the half-life of diazepam when these two drugs are used in combination.

12. When trazodone has been used in combination with digoxin, increased serum digoxin levels have been reported.

13. When trazodone has been used in combination with phenytoin, increased serum phenytoin levels have been reported.

CHAPTER 3

Lithium and Other Mood Stabilizers

Lithium is the most important of the mood-stabilizing drugs, and is the only drug currently approved for the treatment of bipolar disorder. Thus, this chapter will focus primarily on lithium. There are two other classes of mood-stabilizing drugs: the anticonvulsants, including carbamazepine, valproic acid, and clonazepam, and the calcium channel blockers, including verpamamil and diltiazem. Although originally introduced into psychiatry for the treatment of acute mania, mood-stabilizers have also been found to have a prophylactic effect on the course of bipolar disorder (manic-depressive illness). The mood-stabilizing action of these drugs is their ability to prevent the cycling between mania and depression that is the signature of this disease. Aside from their primary use in treating bipolar disorder, the mood-stabilizing drugs are also used for periodic aggressive behavior. Lithium also has a specific use in augmenting the action of antidepressants in antidepressant-resistant depressions.

Before the introduction of lithium, there was no good treatment for bipolar disorder. Bromides, barbiturates, and atropine were not particularly effective. Uncontrolled manic excitement and depressive stupor resulted in high morbidity and mortality. Introduced in the 1930s, electroconvulsive therapy (ECT) was only episodically effective, requiring repeated hospitalizations. It was also a potentially dangerous treatment, because its use had not yet been modified with muscle relaxants and oxygenation. Complications in the form of fractures and brain damage were frequent. The introduction of antipsychotic drugs in the 1950s improved the treatment of mania, but the side effects were severe and the action of these drugs was nonspecific. Some of the symptoms of mania, particularly disturbed thinking, were not touched. Another problem with the use of antipsychotics was their tendency to cause bipolar patients to cycle into depression.

Although lithium was used in the nineteenth century for the treatment of gout, and lithium bromide was used as a sedative and anticonvulsant, the modern story of lithium really begins in 1949 when an Australian physician, John Cade, was searching for a toxin in the urine of manic patients. He discovered that the urine from patients with mania killed rats more often than did urine from controls, and he thought that this was caused by increased urea in mania. Reasoning that uric acid might decrease the toxicity of urea, he chose lithium urate because it was the most soluble urate salt. He believed that the addition of lithium urate or carbonate protected rats from the toxin. When he went on to test lithium on guinea pigs, he was struck with its calming effect. His theory of the antitoxin effect of lithium and his observation that lithium had a quieting behavioral effect in an animal model led Cade to start a clinical trial on 10 manic patients, all of whom responded when treated with lithium. The effectiveness of lithium for the acute treatment of mania was confirmed in Europe. Its usefulness in the prevention of recurrences was studied exhaustively by the Danish psychiatrist, Mogens Schou.

Before the introduction of lithium in the United States, schizophrenia was grossly overdiagnosed. Lithium has an important place in the history of psychiatric nosology because the discovery of its differential effectiveness in manic-depressive illness versus schizophrenia sensitized American psychiatrists to the importance of careful diagnosis and contributed to the demand for a better diagnostic system. From a socioeconomic point of view, the importance of lithium treatment can be appreciated from a study of the impact of lithium in the United States over the 10-year period from 1970 to 1980. Lithium saved approximately 4 billion dollars in medical costs and increased productivity.

The discovery of the mood-stabilizing properties of anticonvulsants has resulted in the development of therapeutic alternatives for the treatment of bipolar and related disorders. It has also stimulated theoretical investigations of possible links between the pathophysiology of bipolar disorder and epileptic phenomena. The parallels between complex partial seizures (temporal lobe epilepsy) and rapid cycling bipolar disorder are particularly striking. Psychiatric theory is borrowing from neurological models of epilepsy (e.g., kindling) to explain other paroxysmal or periodic mental phenomena (aggression, paranoia, panic).

CHEMICAL AND PHARMACOLOGIC PROPERTIES

Lithium

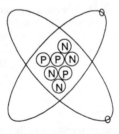

Bohr model of the lithium ion

Lithium is the lightest metal known, having an atomic number of 3 and an atomic weight of 7 (3 protons, 4 neutrons). Only hydrogen and helium are lighter elements. Chemically, it belongs to the same group as sodium, potassium, rubidium, and cesium. The lithium ion has the highest electrical field density of all of the above cations, with which it competes. Its high rate of passage through cell membrane ion channels impedes the influx of the naturally occurring cations. The end result is stabilization of an electrolyte imbalance and thus stabilization of the cell membrane.

Mechanism of Action of Lithium

Lithium has clinical effects on electrolytes, neurotransmitters, receptors, and second messengers. Because there is no unified theory of its mood-stabilizing effect, separate hypotheses have been developed for its antimanic and antidepressant actions. Lithium's antidepressant effect is thought to be due to its ability to increase serotonin and its ability to down-regulate beta receptors. Lithium's antimanic effect may be due to its ability to decrease dopamine receptor supersensitivity, increase cholinergic-muscarinic activity, and inhibit cyclic adenosine monophosphate (AMP) and phosphoinositides.

1. *The ionic competition hypothesis.* Lithium competes with the endogenous cations (sodium, potassium, calcium, and magnesium) in cell membrane ion channels, stabilizing neurotransmitter receptors by correcting an electrolyte imbalance. Neurotransmitters regulating mood are influenced by these cations.

2. *Neurotransmitter hypotheses.* Lithium has effects on serotonin, norepinephrine, gamma-aminobutyric acid (GABA), dopamine, and acetylcholine. These effects suggest several possibilities for lithium's mechanism of action. Lithium increases the activity of serotonin, which would have an antimanic effect if manic patients have supersensitive serotonin receptors. Its serotonergic activity has a direct antidepressant effect and has a synergistic effect when combined with antidepressants. The finding that lithium prevents mood elevation caused by methylphenidate and amphetamine suggests that lithium decreases noradrenergic activity. Also, lithium increases GABA, decreases dopamine, and increases choline.

3. *Receptor hypotheses.* Lithium acts on neurotransmitter receptors. Its ability to decrease dopamine supersensitivity may help account for its antimanic and antipsychotic properties. Lithium has differing effects on α- and β-adrenergic receptors and an affinity for cholinergic-muscarinic receptors.

4. *Second messenger hypotheses.* Two second-messenger systems are thought to be involved with lithium, cyclic AMP and the phosphoinositides. Lithium's ability to inhibit cyclic AMP is related not only to its clinical effects but also to the development of renal and thyroid side effects. Its inhibition of the phosphoinositide system results in the stabilization of neurotransmitters.

Pharmacology of Lithium

Lithium was not introduced into American psychiatry until 1970. This delay was the result of a misguided introduction of lithium as a salt substitute for cardiac patients. Its potential toxicity was not appreciated, and a number of patients died from lithium poisoning. It was this traumatic experience with lithium in American cardiology that resulted in an extremely cautious approach to its reintroduction as a psychiatric drug.

The pharmacokinetics of lithium is straightforward because lithium has no metabolites. The lithium ion is not bound to proteins in the blood or the tissues. The concentration of lithium in the blood is easily and inexpensively measured with flame photometry. Lithium is absorbed rapidly from the gastrointestinal tract when administered by mouth. Peak absorption occurs within an hour or two, and lithium is completely absorbed in 8 hours. Its half-life is about 24 hours and a steady state is reached 5 days after repeated dosing. Lithium is eliminated by the kidneys. In the proximal tubules, 80% of lithium is reabsorbed with sodium and water, and 20% is excreted by the distal tubules. Because lithium is treated by the kidneys as if it were sodium, such sodium depletion as might occur if the patient were to go on a low-salt diet or experience serious vomiting causes retention of lithium and potential toxicity. Lithium has a low therapeutic index, or safety margin, requiring careful clinical and laboratory monitoring. Lithium levels are measured in mEq/L. A useful rule of thumb is that each 300 mg dose raises the lithium plasma level by 0.3 mEq/L. The therapeutic range is generally between 0.5 mEq/L and 1.2 mEq/L. Severe toxicity occurs above 2 mEq/L, and levels above 4 mEq/L are considered life-threatening.

Anticonvulsants

The first widely used anticonvulsant was ECT, which has been used for 50 years for the treatment of depression. Bilateral ECT is also effective in mania. ECT is the most effective treatment for depression and may be the only really effective treatment for some delusional depressions that occur in bipolar disorder. Of course ECT induces seizures, but repeated shocks, as are required in clinical treatment, raise the seizure threshold. In animal models, ECT prevents amygdyla-kindled seizures and has a long-lasting anticonvulsant effect once these seizures have occurred. It has not been shown that ECT's efficacy is due directly to its anticonvulsant effect. There are some plausible alternative hypotheses, which include the theories that seizures cause a nonspecific outpouring of neurotransmitters or that ECT has a direct stimulating effect on the hypothalamus.

The most widely accepted anticonvulsant drugs in psychiatry are carbamazepine, valproic acid, and clonazepam.

Carbamazepine

Carbamazepine (Tegretol) is an iminostilbene derivative, chemically similar to the tricyclic antidepressants. Its carbamyl side chain is essential for its anticonvulsant activity. It is well-established that carbamazepine suppresses kindling. Carbamazepine acts on the benzodiazepine receptor (GABAergic system), the α-adrenergic system, and ion channels. Its α_2-receptor activity is associated with its anti-kindling effect. Its ion-channel activity involves sodium and calcium.

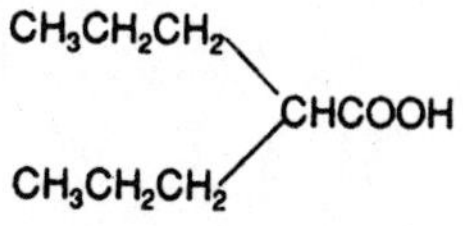

$$CH_3CH_2CH_2 \diagdown$$
$$CHCOOH$$
$$CH_3CH_2CH_2 \diagup$$

Valproic acid

Valproic acid (Depakene) is a simple branched-chain carboxylic acid. It increases GABA functioning and suppresses kindling.

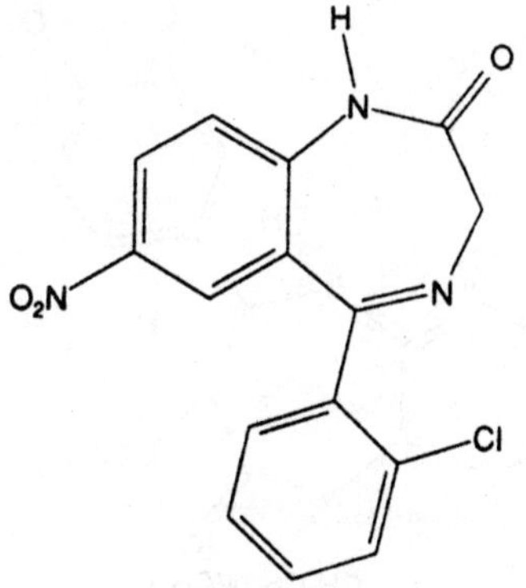

Clonazepam

Clonazepam (Klonopin), a 7-nitrobenzodiazepine derivative, is useful in the treatment of absence (petit mal) and myoclonic seizures. It binds to the benzodiazepine receptor and is serotonergic. It is effective in panic disorder, bipolar disorder, and mania, including secondary mania caused by medical problems (e.g., steroid-induced). There is evidence for both antimanic and antidepressant efficacy, although its antimanic action is much better established and some clinicians believe it can cause depression.

Calcium Channel Blockers

Calcium channel blockers inhibit the movement of calcium ions into cells. Bipolar patients have high cerebrospinal fluid (CSF) calcium when depressed and low calcium CSF levels when manic. ECT, lithium, and verapamil affect concentrations of calcium at the synapse.

Verapamil

Verapamil (Calan) is a benzeneacetonitrile originally introduced as a coronary vasodilator. It is a weak anticonvulsant believed to have a clinically significant antimanic effect.

Diltiazem

Diltiazem (Cardizem) is a benzothiazepine. It may also have antimanic activity.

INDICATIONS FOR USE

Lithium is the drug of choice for bipolar disorder. The diagnosis is made on the basis of a manic episode not explained by a medical cause. Most patients who present with mania go on to have recurrences of mania and depression. Lithium is indicated for the prevention of recurrences of these cyclic mood shifts. An atypical form of this disorder presents with hypomania alternating with major depression and is known as bipolar type II. It also responds to lithium, perhaps less predictably. Some bipolar patients, and especially bipolar II patients, have a seasonal mood disorder that begins in the fall and remits in the spring. Seasonal mood disorder responds to lithium, sometimes in combination with antidepressants and high-intensity light treatment (phototherapy).

Disturbances of mood secondary to medical problems (organic mood syndromes) should be ruled out. The most common causes of organic mood syndromes are drugs and endocrine disorders. Amphetamines, cocaine, and other stimulants (even coffee) can cause a manic syndrome. Endocrine disorders can cause either depression or mania (hyperthyroidism, hypothyroidism; hyperadrenocorticalism, hypoadrenocorticalism). Structural damage to the brain (cerebrovascular accident, multiple sclerosis, infection) may cause either depression or mania.

1. *Manic phase of bipolar disorder.* A typical manic episode is characterized by elevated mood, grandiosity, decreased need for sleep, overtalkativeness, racing thoughts, distractibility, hyperactivity, and poor judgment. Lithium is generally the most effective drug for mania. Because it takes a week or two to begin working, lithium is usually combined with an antipsychotic drug at the start of treatment. Benzodiazepines are sometimes added to control agitation. The anticonvulsant benzodiazepine drug clonazepam is often used. Patients with mild hypomanic syndromes can be treated with lithium or benzodiazepines alone and should not be exposed to antipsychotics because of the risk of tardive dyskinesia.

2. *Depressive phase of bipolar disorder.* A typical major depressive episode is characterized by depressed mood, loss of interest, weight loss, disturbed sleep, psychomotor retardation, fatigue, guilt, loss of interest and enjoyment, impaired concentration, and suicidal ideation. Lithium is effective in decreasing the frequency and severity of the cyclic recurrences of depression in bipolar disorder. If depression occurs during lithium treatment, an antidepressant drug is usually added to lithium. It is particularly important to rule out thyroid disease, because lithium can cause hypothyroidism with associated depression. Monoamine oxidase inhibitors may be effective if the patient fails to respond to tricyclic antidepressants. ECT is extremely effective but is usually reserved for drug-refractory patients.

3. *Maintenance treatment of bipolar disorder.* Bipolar disorder is a chronic illness with exacerbations and remissions. The bipolar patient should generally continue to receive lithium treatment, even after becoming asymptomatic, to avoid a recurrence of a manic or depressive episode. Untreated, the patient may have 10 to 20 episodes in a lifetime and may be at high risk for suicide as well as social and financial catastrophes.

4. *Cyclothymia* is a chronic subsyndromal mood disorder characterized by numerous periods of hypomania and numerous periods of dysthymic depression. Patients with cyclothymia who respond to lithium probably suffer from a forme fruste of bipolar disorder. The mood swings of cyclothymia tend to have a mechanical, predictable quality. Cyclothymic patients misdiagnosed as having borderline personality disorder (a character disorder with labile affect and impulsive behavior) may respond to lithium. Some patients with borderline personality disorder, specifically those with "behavioral dyscontrol" (impulsive aggressiveness or self-harm), have been reported to respond to carbamazepine.

5. *Schizoaffective disorder* is a diagnostic blend of schizophrenia and bipolar disorder. It is divided into bipolar and depressive types. Schizoaffective disorder often responds to lithium combined with an antipsychotic or antidepressant drug. The anticonvulsant carbamazepine is also used in this disorder.

6. *Major depression* is initially treated with antidepressant drugs. Lithium augments responsiveness to antidepressant therapy. With lithium augmentation, the patient with a depression resistant to an antidepressant drug has a two-thirds probability of responding within a day to a month. Carbamazepine is also used for refractory depressions but with much less success.

7. *Schizophrenia* is not an indication for lithium, but lithium may improve the response of some patients to antipsychotic drugs. Because the diagnosis of schizophrenia is inexact and some patients diagnosed as schizophrenic may really be bipolar or schizoaffective, a trial of lithium may be indicated. For example, patients who initially present with an irritable paranoid delusional syndrome may respond to lithium. Patients who have an atypical syndrome reminiscent of mood disorders (i.e., with acute onset, intense disturbance of mood, and/or a family history of mood disorder) should also be considered for a trial on lithium.

8. *Alcohol dependence* secondary to bipolar disorder and other mood disorders is common. Bipolar alcoholics must remain abstinent if they are to benefit from lithium therapy. The use of lithium for the treatment of primary alcoholism is controversial. Although there is evidence that lithium benefits certain alcoholics, it has not become a major treatment for alcoholism.

9. *Late luteal phase disorder* may be diagnosed in patients who present with complaints of severe premenstrual tension syndrome (PMS). It is not known whether lithium is effective in this newly defined syndrome, for which there is a stipulation that major depression is absent. What is known, however, is that many female patients who have a preexisting mood disorder (unipolar as well as bipolar and schizoaffective) have premenstrual exacerbations of their mood disturbances. Lithium alone, or combined with antidepressants or antidepressant–antipsychotic combinations, has been effective in a number of such cases.

10. *Intermittent explosive disorder* is characterized by periodic loss of control of aggressive impulses. It is poorly defined and understood. Of course, patients with bipolar disorder who have lost control and become aggressive should respond to lithium, but they are not considered to belong to this group. However, aggressive patients outside the bipolar spectrum may also respond, suggesting that lithium has a specific anti-aggressive action. Some reports indicate that patients with mental retardation who engage in self-mutilation as well as outwardly aggressive behavior have responded to lithium. The anticonvulsant carbamazepine and the beta blocker propranolol have also been used for aggressive behavior, particularly in patients with neuropsychiatric problems caused by head injuries.

11. *Organic brain syndromes* in which there is aggression or a mood disturbance will sometimes respond to lithium. These include syndromes caused by head trauma, brain tumors, cerebrovascular accidents, postneurosurgical conditions, and dementia. Knowledge in this area is particularly sparse. Patients should be worked up carefully, considered for more conservative treatment, and be informed of the increased risk of neurotoxicity associated with lithium and organicity. Alternatives such as antipsychotics and antidepressants should be considered. In the case of mania or depression secondary to complex partial seizures (temporal lobe epilepsy) the drug of choice is carbamazepine, although many of these patients will require the addition of other drugs

(antipsychotics, antidepressants, antianxiety agents) for satisfactory control of the full range of psychiatric sequelae.

12. *Obsessive compulsive disorder* is treated with antidepressant drugs (clomipramine and fluoxetine have specific antiobsessional activity). The possibility that lithium has an augmenting effect is being researched.

13. *The antiviral effect of lithium* is currently being investigated in herpes simplex and other DNA viruses. Recent use of lithium to treat human immunodeficiency (HIV) infections has not been promising (HIV is an RNA virus). The possibility that a viral infection is involved in the pathophysiology of bipolar disorder or causes a phenocopy has not been ruled out.

GUIDELINES FOR CLINICAL USE OF LITHIUM

Once the patient meets the symptomatic criteria for bipolar disorder, the patient's medical condition should be assessed to determine whether medical problems are causing the syndrome and whether it is medically safe to use lithium and/or other psychiatric drugs to treat it.

1. The diagnostic work-up should include a comprehensive psychiatric and medical history and examination, complete blood count, an extensive metabolic screening battery, thyroid panel, a test for syphilis (preferably FTA-ABS), urinalysis, and, if epilepsy is suspected, a sleep-deprived electroencephalogram with nasopharyngeal leads. If lateralizing signs are present on the neurological examination, a computed axial tomography or magnetic resonance imaging scan is indicated. A history or finding of a static brain lesion might justify neuropsychological testing after the patient's psychiatric condition has been stabilized.

2. The pretreatment work-up is a medical screen to establish the safety of treating the patient with lithium and serves as a baseline for comparison if side effects develop. The standard work-up is a complete blood count, a battery of biochemical tests that should include at least electrolytes, BUN, creatinine (some clinicians order a 24-hour urine for total volume and creatinine clearance), thyroid function tests (thyroid stimulating hormone [TSH], triiodothyronine [T_3], thyroxine [T_4]) and urinalysis. In middle-aged and older patients, an electrocardiogram is also obtained. Patients with preexisting medical problems known to be influenced by lithium (renal disease, thyroid disease, cardiac disease) should be checked by a consultant. Electrolytes must be in balance to avoid lithium toxicity. Impaired kidney functioning requires lower doses of lithium.

3. Treatment of a full manic syndrome should occur in the hospital. Because of the lag time of about 2 weeks between the start of lithium treatment and the beginning of an adequate therapeutic response, an antipsychotic or antianxiety drug is usually prescribed along with lithium. Antipsychotics are indicated for delusions, hallucinations, and aggressive behavior. Benzodiazepines may be sufficient for the pleasantly manic patient. Haldol is the most commonly used antipsychotic drug. Clonazepam and lorazepam are commonly used benzodiazepines. Clonazepam has a theoretical advantage because of its anticonvulsant activity. Lorazepam has a practical advantage because of its very short half-life, allowing for rapid dose adjustment, and its availability in intramuscular (IM) form. Unlike diazepam, lorazepam is reliably absorbed after IM injection.

4. The starting dose of lithium is 300 mg two or three times a day. The dose is then increased gradually while the patient's clinical status and lithium level are monitored. The usual lithium level for acute mania is 0.8 to 1.2 mEq/L. Lithium levels above 1.5 mEq/L are seldom required. Younger adults and larger patients tend to require higher doses. Older patients, children, and the medically ill tend to require lower doses. In the average floridly manic adult, the usual therapeutic dose range is 1200 to 1800 mg for initial control. However, some patients will require higher doses. In geriatric patients the usual range is 300 mg to 900 mg. Lithium levels should be obtained twice a week until the patient and the lithium level are both stable. Because it takes 5 days to reach a steady state, it is pointless to adjust the dose more than once a week. Of course, it is rational to change the dose more often for clinical reasons (e.g., evident toxicity). Failure to respond at 1.5 mEq/L for a few weeks should prompt a review of the diagnosis. If the clinician maintains the conviction that the patient is manic and wants to avoid antipsychotic drugs, an anticonvulsant, usually carbamazepine, is added. Some clinicians reduce the dose of lithium to avoid a toxic reaction to the drug combination. Antipsychotic and antianxiety drugs are also effective in treatment-resistant patients. The ideal is to have the patient in full remission on lithium alone, but that is not always possible. Once the patient and the lithium level are stable, the frequency of blood testing is reduced. Whenever a crisis develops, whether medical or psychiatric, a lithium level should be obtained. This can help to determine whether the patient is toxic, undermedicated, or noncompliant. Special care should be taken with patients who are medically ill, have brain disease, or are elderly, all of whom should receive less aggressive treatment in order to avoid toxicity.

5. The maintenance dose is determined by what is found, through trial and error, to be the lowest effective dose. It is common for the patient to require less lithium after remission. This is indicated by a rising lithium level on a steady dose. The dose of lithium should be adjusted downward to avoid toxicity. Most patients have a particular dosage and lithium level that works for them most of the time. Usually this is a dosage between 900 and 1200 mg and a level between 0.5 mEq/L and 1.0 mEq/L.

During outpatient treatment the patient may need to take more lithium during periods of exacerbation, particularly if the symptoms are manic. Breakthrough depressions are usually handled with the addition of an antidepressant drug. There is a possibility that the antidepressant drug bupropion exerts a prophylactic effect for bipolar disorder. It may be effective both for rapid-cycling bipolar disorder and for prophylaxis of slow-cyclers. Severe or intractable mania can be treated by adding carbamazepine or clonazepam. Mild manic symptoms may be treated with almost any benzodiazepine, although the atypical benzodiazepine alprazolam should be avoided because of the theoretical possibility that its antidepressant activity could cause the mania to worsen. Manic breakthroughs presenting with insomnia can sometimes be aborted with flurazepam or clonazepam. In general, when the patient becomes symptomatic, the target symptom should determine the type of drug chosen. For brief periods of time, it is perfectly rational to add an antipsychotic, antianxiety, or antidepressant drug, particularly if it is known that these measures have worked in the past for a given patient.

Although not standard practice, patients are being treated successfully with a single daily dose of lithium. Theoretically, this may reduce noncompliance and reduce the risk of renal complications.

Patients should be educated about the right way to have their lithium level determined. The test is standardized at 12 hours following the last dose. If the patient takes the morning dose of lithium just before the blood is drawn, the test will be invalidated. Usually, the most convenient way for the patient to have a lithium level done is to take the last dose at night and have the blood level drawn 12 hours later, before the morning dose of lithium. Outpatients who are clinically stable on maintenance lithium therapy should have levels drawn monthly. Very reliable and stable patients may be tested less often, perhaps once every 2 to 3 months.

6. The psychological management of the bipolar patient is just as important as the pharmacologic management of his or her disease. Bipolar patients, particularly those who have had a dramatic response to lithium, tend to deny the need for maintenance treatment. This is often based on their experience of being treated with a transparent drug that has allowed them to become completely asymptomatic. It has been suggested that bipolar patients have impaired right-hemisphere functioning and that their denial may share its etiology with the denial seen in neurological patients with right-hemisphere lesions. A related problem is that many bipolar patients do not observe their own mood swings. Proper psychological management early in treatment may spell the difference between success and failure in the long run.

The first step in the psychological management of the bipolar patient is enlisting the patient in a lifelong program of treatment that may involve a psychotherapeutic, didactic, or family approach along with lithium therapy. For example, it may be helpful to have a family member discuss the warning signals that preceded the patient's manic and depressive episodes and to have the relative work with both the patient and the psychiatrist to help avoid a relapse.

The clinician must be prepared for the time when the patient decides to try to go without lithium. In the absence of a laboratory test for the disease, this may represent healthy reality testing on the patient's part and may result (after relapse) in a commitment to treatment. Because catastrophes can occur, every effort should be made before discharge from the hospital to educate the patient and family about the chronic nature of bipolar disorder. Because of the high risk of recurrence, which is associated with a high degree of morbidity and mortality, maintenance treatment should be initiated after the first manic episode if there is a family history of bipolar disorder or if it is judged that a second episode might be catastrophic.

Thus, psychological management early in treatment should focus on educating the patient and the family about the chronicity of bipolar disorder and developing a therapeutic relationship that motivates the patient to stay in treatment. Later in treatment, patients often need help in discriminating between changes in mood that can be explained by neurotic reactions to stressful life events, episodes of illness that are triggered directly by stress, and episodes that seem to be part of the natural history of the disorder itself, such as seasonal exacerbations. Stressful life events may trigger manic or depressive episodes, and psychotherapy aimed at avoidance of avoidable stress and awareness of personal vulnerabilities can be an important part of the overall treatment. Discussion with a reliable member of the family is often helpful in understanding the interaction of problems in living with episodes of illness.

Based on twin and family studies, there is indisputable evidence of a genetic factor in bipolar disorder. In spite of its heritability, there is no laboratory test to make the diagnosis. There are probably several genetic subtypes complicating the search for a biological marker. A family history of bipolar disorder and a familial response to lithium are useful data and, when combined with a good clinical response to lithium in the patient, are as close as currently possible to confirming the diagnosis. Genetic counseling can be reassuring to the patient and family if the patient's response has been satisfactory. A frank discussion of the risk to blood relatives might lead to earlier recognition and treatment of bipolar disorder. This might lead in turn to less morbidity and a reduction in the high suicide rate of bipolar patients.

Bipolar disorder is associated with creativity and is especially common in writers. There is little evidence that lithium actually reduces creativity, although in some instances a reduction in the lithium level has resulted in better acceptance by the creative patient.

SIDE EFFECTS OF LITHIUM

Early in treatment nausea, loose stools, increased thirst, a metallic taste, tremor, fatigue, and polyuria are common. These symptoms usually abate with time. The long-term side effects are dose-related and correlate fairly well with lithium levels. Weight gain, which does not appear to correlate with dose, is common and should be treated with diet and exercise. Although nausea and vomiting may occur at therapeutic levels, they may be warning signs of impending toxicity, which usually occurs at levels above 1.5 mEq/L. A definitive review of the most common misconceptions about lithium side effects has recently been published by Mogens Schou. Detailed and updated information on the side effects of lithium are available from the *Lithium Library*, an on-line data base at the University of Wisconsin, and the derivative handbook, *Lithium Encyclopedia for Clinical Practice*.

1. *Gastrointestinal*. Complaints of nausea and loose stools are common during the first week of treatment. Some patients complain of a metallic taste in the mouth. Less frequently, abdominal pain, vomiting, and diarrhea may occur. These side effects coincide with plasma lithium peaks, which occur after rapid absorption. Gastrointestinal side effects are usually mild and diminish as patients adapt to the absorptive peaks of the drug. A reduction in dose is not usually indicated. Prescribing lithium to be taken after meals tends to avoid or ameliorate these effects. If this measure is not effective, a slow-release preparation (Lithobid; Eskalith CR) may help. Patients who take lithium and vomit from an influenza-like viral illness may develop an electrolyte imbalance causing toxicity. Patients on maintenance lithium therapy should be advised to stop taking lithium if vomiting occurs.

2. *Neurological*. Early in treatment patients may complain of fatigue, muscle weakness, and malaise. Frequently they will have a fine resting tremor noticeable in the fingers and affecting handwriting. This tremor may disappear or may persist at therapeutic levels. Lowering the dose of lithium may eliminate the problem if the patient does not relapse. The tremor can often be eliminated with propranolol, 20 to 80 mg daily in divided doses. Patients

treated with propranolol should be watched for depression. Beta blockers (atenolol, metoprolol) that have a preferential effect on β_1-adrenoreceptors do not cross the blood-brain barrier as readily as propranolol and may be less likely to cause depression. Toxic side effects have been occasionally seen at therapeutic lithium levels. These include ataxia, dysarthria, extrapyramidal symptoms, confusion, muscle twitching, and choreoathetotic movements. Symptoms of lithium toxicity must be closely monitored. A lithium level should be drawn immediately and lithium stopped or reduced.

3. *Kidney.* It is common for polyuria (diuresis) to take place in the first few days of treatment. Polyuria and polydipsia are usually mild and well-tolerated but may continue to occur if the maintenance dose is high. Rarely, severe polyuria and polydipsia (lithium-induced nephrogenic diabetes insipidus) occurs at therapeutic levels. It is caused by lithium's interference with the action of antidiuretic hormone (ADH, vasopressin) on adenylate cyclase, which results in a reduction of water reabsorption in the distal nephron. It may cause renal damage if not treated and is a justification for switching to carbamazepine as an alternative drug. However, treatment with a potassium-sparing diuretic, amiloride (5 to 10 mg bid), has shown good results. Desmopressin acetate (DDAVP) may also be effective, but it requires intradermal injections or intranasal application. Studies of long-term renal side effects of lithium have demonstrated pathological changes in the kidney including a decrease in renal concentrating ability, decreased creatinine clearance, focal nephron atrophy, and interstitial fibrosis. Prudence dictates periodic monitoring of creatinine levels (at least twice a year) and consultation with a nephrologist if creatinine levels climb abnormally high. Some clinicians also recommend a yearly 24-hour urine creatine clearance, because this is a more sensitive indicator of renal function. A steady rise in the lithium level at a constant dose of lithium is a good reason to check the patient's creatinine level. An overdose can cause irreversible kidney damage and require lifelong dialysis.

4. *Heart.* Lithium is well-tolerated by the cardiovascular system. ECG changes similar to those seen with hypokalemia may be seen. Flattening and inversion of the T wave are the most common changes. They are benign and reversible and are thought to be caused by lithium displacing intracellular potassium. Rarely, cardiac arrhythmias have first appeared with lithium treatment. Lithium may depress the pacemaker function of the sinus node, and sinus node arrhythmias may occur.

5. *Thyroid.* Hypothyroidism, with or without the development of goiter, occurs in 5% of patients taking lithium. The most sensitive indicator of thyroid function is TSH, which should be ordered at least once a year. T_3 and T_4 should also be obtained. Because of its sensitivity, TSH should be substantially elevated before treatment is contemplated. Because hypothyroidism commonly presents with depression and interferes with the action of antidepressants, it is important to check thyroid function if a bipolar patient becomes depressed. Other warning symptoms are weight gain, hair loss, and complaints of memory impairment. Hypothyroidism is easily treated with thyroid replacement therapy and does not require discontinuation of lithium. T_3-triiodothyronine has been used as an adjunctive treatment for treatment-resistant bipolar depression, and T_4-thyroxine has been used in combination with lithium for rapid-cycling bipolar patients and may be effective even in chemically euthyroid patients. Thyroid treatment is monitored with serial T_3, T_4

and TSH levels. Women and patients with a history of thyroid disease are at greatest risk for lithium-induced hypothyroidism.

6. *Edema*. Pretibial and hand edema may be caused by increased aldosterone levels causing sodium retention. Edema may disappear spontaneously. If it is persistent and troublesome, cautious treatment with spironolactone is usually safe and effective.

7. *Weight gain*. This is a common complication of lithium treatment and an important cause of noncompliance. A weight gain of 30 lbs. is not uncommon. A weight-reducing diet (not salt restricted) is usually effective. The cause of the weight gain is not known, but it may be due to altered carbohydrate metabolism. Other possible causes are the drinking of high-calorie beverages because of polydipsia, edema, and lithium-induced hypothyroidism. If the patient wants to go on a programmed or packaged diet, it is important to review it to make sure the patient is not inadvertently salt-restricted.

8. *Leukocytosis*. The white blood count may reach 20,000 without ill effect. Benign granulocytosis has also been reported. This phenomenon reverses if lithium is discontinued but, because it is a benign event, is not a reason to stop lithium treatment. It is important mainly because it may cause unwarranted alarm and an unnecessary workup if another physician involved in caring for the patient does not know that the patient is taking lithium. Lithium has been used with variable success in treating neutropenia caused by cancer chemotherapy. It seems to be a reliable treatment for carbamazepine-induced neutropenia.

9. *Skin*. Lithium can cause or exacerbate acne and sometimes exacerbates psoriasis and causes rashes. Acne and psoriasis should be treated with the standard methods. Rashes sometimes respond to antihistamines or topical steroids. They may remit spontaneously.

10. *Pregnancy*. Lithium should not be used during the first trimester of pregnancy and must be used with caution during the last two trimesters (see the section on Use in Pregnancy and Lactation).

LITHIUM TOXICITY

Toxicity with lithium use does not generally occur until the level reaches 2 mEq/L, but some individuals are hypersensitive to lithium and develop toxic symptoms at therapeutic levels. Lithium toxicity occurring at therapeutic doses is commonly due to a drug-drug interaction with a thiazide diuretic. Thiazide diuretics cause lithium retention and raise the lithium level. Other common causes of toxicity are impaired renal function, salt restriction, and dehydration. Lithium has been reported to increase the likelihood of post-ECT delirium.

1. Thiazide diuretics should receive special attention because they are widely used to treat hypertension. If the patient must be on one, the dose of lithium should be reduced by 50% and carefully titrated with frequent monitoring of the lithium level.

2. Organic brain syndromes present the greatest constitutional risk of developing lithium toxicity, as does advanced age. Patients with schizophrenia may also be more prone to develop lithium toxicity.

3. Drug-drug interactions causing lithium toxicity have been reported in patients taking combinations of lithium with antipsychotics, anticonvulsants, and calcium channel blockers.

Nonsteroidal antiinflammatory agents, with the exceptions of aspirin, sulindac (Clinoril), and flurbiprofen (Ansaid), have been associated with increased lithium levels. Drugs to avoid include indomethacin (Indocin) and ibuprofen (Motrin).

Angiotensin-converting enzyme inhibitors have been reported to increase lithium levels. These include captopril (Capoten), enalapril (Vasotec), and lisinopril (Prinivil).

4. Clinical observation is more sensitive than the lithium level in the detection of lithium toxicity. If toxicity is suspected, lithium should be withheld and a lithium level obtained. Patients should be educated about the early signs of toxicity, which are usually gastrointestinal, such as nausea, diarrhea, and vomiting. The new development of a tremor or incoordination is also an early indication.

5. Neurological signs usually occur at the intermediate stage of toxicity, beginning with lethargy, drowsiness, dysarthria, blurred vision, ataxia, coarse tremor, muscle twitching, and fasciculations. In advanced stages of lithium toxicity, the patient may have delirium, nystagmus, myoclonic movements, hyperactive deep tendon reflexes, Babinski reflex, choreoathetoid movements, rigidity, and seizures. The EEG shows diffuse slowing. Untreated, severe toxicity will ultimately lead to stupor, coma, and death. Permanent brain damage may follow serious lithium intoxication. Dementia, choreoathetosis, and cerebellar ataxia have been reported.

6. The treatment of lithium toxicity consists of discontinuation of lithium (enough in mild cases), reestablishment of normal electrolyte balance, general supportive measures and, in serious cases, dialysis. Treatment of an overdose with gastric lavage may prevent toxicity from developing. This may be particularly effective with the slow-release preparations.

DRUG INTERACTIONS

Most of the drug–drug interactions are covered in the preceding section on lithium toxicity.

1. Drugs that lower the lithium level include mannitol, urea, acetazolamide (Diamox), aminophylline, theophylline, and sodium bicarbonate.

2. Lithium prolongs the action of the muscle relaxants pancuronium bromide (Pavulon) and succinylcholine (Anectine). Lithium should be discontinued if these agents are to be used before surgery or ECT.

ALTERNATIVES TO LITHIUM

Lithium is effective in 67% of bipolar patients, leaving a sizeable number of patients with no therapeutic response or in partial remission. The choice of an alternative or adjunctive drug depends initially on whether the patient is currently in a manic or a depressive state. Mania can be treated with benzodiazepines, anticonvulsants, antipsychotics, or calcium channel blockers. Although many patients who do not respond to lithium can be treated with antipsychotics combined with antidepressants, most clinicians are trying to avoid antipsychotics because of the higher risk of tardive dyskinesia in bipolar patients. Another problem with the antipsychotic-antidepressant combination is that it tends to destabilize mood by increasing the frequency of cycling. ECT is effective in both mania and depression and has a high probability of working in drug-refractory cases, but its effectiveness as a maintenance treatment for bipolar disorder has not been established.

Anticonvulsants

The psychiatric efficacy of *carbamazepine* was first observed when patients taking it for episodes of trigeminal neuralgia and complex partial seizures experienced a dramatic improvement in mood. Evidence of its mood-stabilizing properties are reports that suggest that it is especially useful for patients who cycle more than three times a year (rapid-cyclers) and that it is an effective substitute for lithium as a prophylactic agent in bipolar disorder. Carbamazepine is used as an adjunctive drug with lithium for lithium-refractory mania. Its efficacy as an antidepressant is less well documented, but it has an established use as a substitute for lithium-resistant or intolerant patients for both acute mania and prophylaxis of bipolar disorder. The time course of its action in mania is similar to lithium and in depression is similar to a tricyclic antidepressant.

It is not known whether the efficacy of carbamazepine and other anticonvulsants in bipolar disorder is due to their anticonvulsant activity or to some other mechanism. A theory which attempts to explain the action of carbamazepine hypothesizes a continuum between frank epilepsy with convulsive seizures at one extreme, various epileptic equivalent states (subseizures, subictal seizures, paraepileptic states) and rapid-cycling bipolar disorder in between, and slow-cycling bipolar disorder at the other extreme. A theory of "kindling" or irritative, destabilizing buildup of seizure-like activity in the limbic system has been proposed. However, there is not much clinical evidence for this theory and, in fact, refractory patients who present with epileptoid phenomena (e.g., olfactory hallucinations) do not seem to do better on carbamazepine. Carbamazepine has benzodiazepine receptor (GABA) activity, as well as effects on the α-adrenergic system and ion channels. Its α_2-receptor activity is associated with its antikindling effect. Its benzodiazepine receptor activity probably involves calcium rather than chloride channels, and it is believed to stabilize sodium channels.

The most common *side effects* of carbamazepine are rashes, dizziness, drowsiness, and ataxia. The therapeutic range is broader than in epilepsy, from 4 to 12 μg/mL. The patient's clinical response is the best indicator of appropriate dosage, but blood levels are useful in checking for toxicity and for compliance. Carbamazepine is associated with a risk of aplastic anemia and agranulocytosis, but the risk is quite low (1 in 125,000). It commonly causes a benign neutropenia. Serious neutropenias are reversible with lithium. The patient should be started on 100 to 200 mg bid, with a slow increase in dosage to avoid side effects. Because carbamazepine induces hepatic enzymes, patients commonly develop tolerance within a few weeks, the blood level goes down, and it may be necessary to increase the dose.

Common drug interactions that cause increased blood levels of carbamazepine and potential toxicity occur with the antibiotic erythromycin and its chemical relatives, the calcium channel blockers verapamil and diltiazem, cimetidine (Tagamet), isoniazid, and the narcotic analgesic propoxyphene (Darvon). Carbamazepine causes a decrease in the blood levels of antipsychotic drugs (especially haloperidol) and birth control pills. Carbamazepine should be avoided in pregnancy because of its teratogenic effects.

Valproic acid may be effective for acute treatment and prophylaxis of bipolar patients who fail on carbamazepine. The mechanism of action appears to be its ability to increase GABA. The dose range is 250 mg two to four times a day. Side effects include tremor, alopecia, gastrointestinal distress, and weight gain. Severe liver toxicity has been reported. In pregnancy, it is associated with a high risk of spina bifida. Blood levels are less reliable with valproic acid than with carbamazepine.

Clonazepam is used chiefly for its antimanic effects. Because it has a benzodiazepine structure, it is less toxic than the other anticonvulsants when used in combination with other psychiatric drugs. The starting dose is 0.5 mg two or three times a day, and it is titrated up to 6 mg daily. However, some patients will require higher doses. Its mechanism of action appears to involve chloride ion channels. It is not known whether its effectiveness is due to its antianxiety effect or to its anticonvulsant activity. It is less toxic than an antipsychotic for the treatment of mania, but its usefulness in the maintenance treatment of bipolar disorder is yet to be determined, and its antidepressant efficacy is not well-established. It has been demonstrated to be effective in the treatment of panic disorder. The main side effect of clonazepam is oversedation.

Calcium Channel Blockers

Verapamil may be effective in mania when the patient fails to respond to lithium or an anticonvulsant drug. It does not appear to have antidepressant properties and may cause depression. It should still be regarded as an investigational drug. *Diltiazem* may also have antimanic activity that may be useful when conventional methods fail.

USE IN PREGNANCY AND LACTATION

The literature on lithium is replete with warnings about the risk of cardiac malformations in the first trimester of pregnancy. Abnormalities of the tricuspid valve (e.g., Ebstein's malformation) have been the most common cardiac anomalies reported. Although the risk is real, the degree of risk is not known, because the research is based to a large extent on a lithium registry that probably underreports normal outcomes. Most women on lithium deliver normal babies. Cardiac malformations occur in 2% of all babies. The percentage of cardiac malformations in lithium babies is unknown.

Under the circumstances, it should be assumed that lithium is teratogenic. The patient should stop taking lithium before attempting conception and should not take it during the first trimester. Carbamazepine is not a good substitute for lithium in this situation because it, too, is probably teratogenic. Antipsychotics and antidepressants, on the other hand, are relatively safe in pregnancy. ECT is safe and effective in both mania and depression. For patients with mania, clonazepam is another possibility. Lithium can be given during the last two trimesters of pregnancy if there are strong indications for its use.

Childbirth may precipitate lithium toxicity because the renal clearance of lithium increases markedly during pregnancy and falls off rapidly at delivery. A patient who is on lithium should have the dose reduced 1 week before delivery and stopped when labor begins. Lithium should be restarted as soon as the patient becomes physiologically stable in the postpartum period to prevent postpartum mania or depression, which are common (up to 40%) in bipolar patients.

Lithium may cause neonatal distress, that is, a floppy, hypotonic baby with a slowed heart rate, cyanosis, and a low Apgar score. Neonatal toxicity reverses within a few days with supportive treatment.

Since lithium is present in breast milk at about one half the serum concentration, babies born to mothers taking lithium should not be breastfed.

USE IN THE ELDERLY

The use of mood-stabilizing drugs in a geriatric patient follows the general principle of geriatric pharmacology that emphasizes altered pharmacokinetics and pharmacodynamics in old age. The practice of using lower doses and blood levels of drugs and titrating very slowly reflects the clinician's need to adapt to the elderly patient's decreased metabolism and increased receptor sensitivity. Failure to make this adaptation may result in side effects that can eventuate in anything from delirium to hip fractures.

Bipolar patients grow old and require continued treatment, and late-onset bipolar disorder is more common than previously believed. There is a tendency for mania in this age group to present as a dementiform confusional state, and the clinician who is not diagnostically astute will miss a treatment opportunity. Geriatric patients are susceptible to secondary mania, which should be treated etiologically when it is feasible.

Lithium's prophylactic efficacy is undiminished in the geriatric bipolar patient, although the presence of dementia or parkinsonism may increase its toxicity. Maintenance treatment should be tried with lithium levels lower than the 0.7 to 0.8 mEq/L average used in the healthy young adult. The range from 0.4 mEq/L to 0.6 mEq/L is just as effective and safer. An even lower dose of lithium (levels of 0.4 mEq/L or less) is effective for lithium augmentation of antidepressants. The initial dose of lithium should be 300 mg. The dose should not be increased for a week, and not until after a lithium level has been obtained.

Carbamazepine may be useful along with lithium for refractory cases, especially for rapid-cycling patients. It is also a recognized substitute for lithium in patients with impaired renal functioning or those taking diuretics. The dose range in geriatric patients is 300 to 900 mg/d.

Neuroleptics are still used as a last resort in patients for whom lithium and carbamazepine are not effective or safe.

CHAPTER 4

Antianxiety Drugs

For all practical purposes, the psychopharmacology of anxiety is the psychopharmacology of the benzodiazepines. These drugs are also used to treat the most common types of insomnia. There are two important atypical antianxiety drugs: alprazolam (Xanax), a triazolobenzodiazepine, which has both antianxiety and antidepressant (and, therefore, antipanic) activity; and buspirone (BuSpar), a prototype of the azaspirones, a new class of antianxiety agents thought to produce less sedation that the benzodiazepines.

Alcohol is the oldest, and most dangerous, antianxiety drug. Physicians prescribed alcohol for centuries for its anesthetic, hypnotic (anti-insomnia), and antianxiety properties. It is likely that alcohol was used for these purposes long before the profession of medicine came into existence.

Serious complications similar to those seen with alcohol use, including tolerance, dependence, and withdrawal, are associated with drugs that were used as anxiolytics and hypnotics before the introduction of the benzodiazepines, most notably the barbiturates and meprobamate. Unfortunately the complications caused by these sedative–hypnotic compounds have created unwarranted fears about benzodiazepines. Guilt by association has led to fear of treating disorders that are severely disabling and potentially life-threatening.

Unlike their predecessors, the benzodiazepines have relatively low abuse potential in properly diagnosed patients and are relatively safe when taken in overdose if not combined with alcohol or barbiturate-like compounds. The functional impairment resulting from anxiety disorders, although widely thought to be minimal, is in fact associated with a substantial lifetime risk of suicide. Anxiety disorders appear to exist on a continuum with depressive disorders. If an untreated anxiety disorder is allowed to progress to a major depression, the lifetime suicide risk goes up. For example, the lifetime risk of suicide attempt in the general population is 1%, in patients with panic disorder it is 7%, and in panic disorder with major depression it is 26%. Other disorders associated with untreated anxiety are alcoholism and various medical problems (peptic ulcer disease, cardiovascular disease, irritable bowel syndrome, neurodermatitis).

The coexistence of benzodiazepines and antidepressants has created difficult nosological challenges. For example, although panic disorder is classified as an anxiety disorder, it responds best to antidepressant drugs. The same is true with obsessive compulsive disorder. At the same time, major depression is sometimes followed by the development of generalized anxiety disorder, and bipolar disorder can sometimes be treated with benzodiazepines. The diagnostic nomenclature will eventually have to take into account the existence of (1) discrete nosological entities and (2) the relationships between them. This has already been appreciated with the invention of the term "schizoaffective." Whether it will be followed by terms linking anxiety with depression, mania, and other well-established entities remains to be seen.

During the nineteenth and early twentieth centuries bromide salts were used as antianxiety agents. By the 1930s "bromide intoxication," a form of delirium, was a recognized side effect, which led to a decline in the use of bromides in medicine. In the late 1800s two compounds similar to alcohol, chloral hydrate and paraldehyde, were used to treat insomnia. Chloral hydrate is still sometimes used for this purpose. Paraldehyde, which was once the drug of choice for the treatment of alcohol withdrawal, has been replaced by the benzodiazepines. The barbiturates came into use in the early part of the twentieth century and were widely used for the treatment of anxiety and insomnia. However, by the 1950s, problems with tolerance, addiction, and withdrawal became apparent. The search for new agents led to the introduction of meprobamate (Miltown) and its congeners, all of which turned out to have the same problems as the barbiturates: tolerance, dependence, alcohol-like withdrawal syndrome, depression, and a high risk of death when taken in overdose.

With the introduction of chlordiazepoxide (Librium) in 1960, a new era in the pharmacologic treatment of anxiety and insomnia began. Chlordiazepoxide was the first drug of the benzodiazepine class to be introduced into medical practice. Since 1960 several other benzodiazepines have been marketed. Because of the greater safety and efficacy of the benzodiazepines, the older agents have become obsolete. The benzodiazepines are therefore the drugs of choice in the treatment of anxiety and insomnia. They are among the most frequently prescribed drugs in the world.

Because of the abuse potential of the benzodiazepines, there has been some controversy regarding their prescription. For example, New York State now requires a triplicate prescription form for benzodiazepines (the same type of form used in prescribing narcotics) to monitor their use more effectively. The benzodiazepines can be abused by susceptible individuals (e.g., alcoholics and other patients with a history of drug abuse) and should not be prescribed in those instances. However, studies have shown that patients with anxiety disorders (without a concurrent drug abuse problem) do not tend to abuse these drugs and, in fact, may take less than the prescribed dose.

Up to 10% of the population suffers from an anxiety disorder, but individuals with anxiety disorders are often not effectively treated. It has been estimated that only one third of patients with anxiety disorders receive treatment and that two thirds of those who do receive treatment receive inadequate treatment. Many cases are not properly diagnosed. Others are undertreated because of concerns about drug abuse. Proper treatment of any illness requires making an accurate diagnosis and then instituting an effective treatment regimen. Benzodiazepines should not be withheld from those patients who would benefit from them. Nor should they be prescribed for individuals likely to abuse them.

Much of the concern about benzodiazepine dependence reflects a lack of appreciation of the difference between (1) dependence on a drug that restores functioning and (2) dependence on a drug that impairs functioning. When properly used, benzodiazepines effectively control anxiety and restore normal functioning to the individual. Thus, patients with anxiety disorders function better with a benzodiazepine. When any drug (including a benzodiazepine) is used in an abusive pattern, functioning is invariably impaired. This important distinction can assist the clinician in the appropriate prescription of benzodiazepines.

Long-term use of benzodiazepines tends to result in tolerance for sedative side effects but not for antianxiety effects, and therefore it does not result in an escalation of dosage. Psychiatric patients with chronic anxiety disorders who take therapeutic doses of benzodiazepines for long periods of time should not be confused with addicted individuals who take high doses of benzodiazepines illicitly, often in combination with other drugs, to "get high."

Proper prescription requires careful diagnosis and regular followup. The ideal patient has a circumscribed anxiety problem and would rather not take a drug. Patients who should not take benzodiazepines include patients with character disorders (e.g., borderline personality disorder) and a history of drug abuse and those who have previously abused benzodiazepines and are unusually anxious to receive them.

CHEMICAL AND PHARMACOLOGIC PROPERTIES
OF BENZODIAZEPINES

The pharmacologic differences between the benzodiazepines are the result of modifications of a nuclear tricyclic structure consisting of a benzene ring (**A**), a diazepine ring (**B**), and a 5-aryl ring (**C**).

Benzodiazepine structure

The benzodiazepines have many different pharmacologic actions, including sedative, hypnotic, antianxiety, anticonvulsant, and muscle-relaxant properties. Benzodiazepine receptors (stereospecific recognition sites for benzodiazepines) were discovered in the rat brain in 1977 and in the human brain in 1978. Although they have been found in a number of other vertebrate species, they have not been found in invertebrates, suggesting that their function is highly evolved. The existence of the benzodiazepine receptor suggests that there are endogenous benzodiazepines. The antianxiety action of the benzodiazepine drugs suggests that endogenous benzodiazepines were evolved as fear-regulating agents. This in turn suggests a modulating function in relationship to the fight-or-flight response and a relationship to its neuroanatomic basis, the noradrenergic system. The densest collection of benzodiazepine receptors in the brain is found in the locus ceruleus, which is also the site of origin of the noradrenergic system. Thus, the greatest density of benzodiazepine receptors and the greatest collection of brain norepinephrine are in the same place. It is plausible to speculate that their close proximity serves a regulatory function.

As early as 1975 it was known that benzodiazepines could enhance the activity of the endogenous inhibitory neurotransmitter gamma-aminobutyric acid (GABA). In 1978 Tallman et al. found that GABA increased the affinity of benzodiazepines to the benzodiazepine receptor, demonstrating a functional link between benzodiazepines and GABA. In 1980, Tallman and Paul et al. published a paper showing that binding of benzodiazepines to the benzodiazepine receptor was also enhanced by chloride and bromide ions, suggesting that a chloride ion channel was also involved in the actions of benzodiazepines.

The current theory of the mechanism of action of the benzodiazepines can be summarized as follows. Benzodiazepines enhance the activity of GABA, the primary inhibitory neurotransmitter in the brain. Benzodiazepine and GABA receptors are closely linked. GABA binds to the GABA receptor, a process that produces a conformational change that opens chloride ion channels in the postsynaptic cell membrane. This hyperpolarizes these neurons and decreases their firing rate. The decreased firing rate reduces anxiety. Benzodiazepines bind to the benzodiazepine receptor. The benzodiazepine receptor is connected to the GABA receptor and a chloride ion channel in what is known as the benzodiazepine-GABA receptor complex. This macromolecule opens the chloride ion channel further, causing further hyperpolarization of the postsynaptic neuron, decreasing its firing rate even more, and resulting in a further reduction in anxiety. It is not known to what extent other neurotransmitters (such as serotonin) might be involved in the regulation of fear and anxiety. What does seem to be known is that benzodiazepines act in concert with GABA and a chloride ion channel to reduce anxiety.

Clinically, the benzodiazepines have several advantages over older antianxiety and hypnotic agents. Their antianxiety effect is more specific and can be achieved with less sedation than with previously developed drugs. They can be used within a wide therapeutic range with a high margin of safety. They are rarely lethal when taken in overdose unless combined with other drugs. Hepatic microsomal enzyme induction is not clinically significant. Thus, they do not interfere with the metabolism of other drugs taken concurrently. Tolerance to benzodiazepines develops slowly, in contrast to tolerance to meprobamate and the barbiturates (with the exception of phenobarbital).

Although physiological addiction can occur with the benzodiazepines, it generally requires the use of high doses over several months' time. Withdrawal syndromes following prolonged use of these agents are also less severe than those associated with the barbiturates and meprobamate, and they are less frequently associated with seizures.

Of all the agents presently used as hypnotics, these agents appear to interfere least with normal physiological sleep. There is less suppression of rapid eye movement (REM) sleep and less REM rebound after withdrawal. Stage 4 (delta) sleep is decreased by benzodiazepines, but this may be compensated for by an increase in the duration of other non-REM sleep stages. Stage 4 sleep returns to normal after discontinuation of the benzodiazepines.

The biggest problem with this class of drugs is habituation or psychological dependence. This problem appears to be more associated with patients who have severe character disorders and who are already polydrug abusers. In other patients, slow tapering of the benzodiazepines rarely results in clinically significant problems unless, of course, the patient needs the drug for the treatment of a chronic anxiety disorder. It is important here to distinguish between dependence as an artifact of drug use and dependence as a reflection of a persistent disease state. The latter is an indication for continued treatment.

The main differences between the benzodiazepines are their pharmacokinetic properties. For example, oxazepam and lorazepam have shorter half-lives and no active metabolites. The other benzodiazepines have longer half-lives, active metabolites, and tend to accumulate. Thus oxazepam and lorazepam may be especially useful in treating elderly patients, those with impaired liver function, and other patients in whom drug accumulation is undesirable. A steady state is reached at about five times the half-life of the drug. It takes diazepam 7 to 10 days to reach a steady state, whereas lorazepam reaches a steady state in 2 to 3 days. Oxazepam is usually prescribed to be taken three or four times a day because of its short half-life. Lorazepam is usually taken two or three times a day. Alprazolam should be taken two to four times a day. The other benzodiazepines should be initially taken two or three times a day until a steady state is reached. Then the dose can be shifted to a once- or twice-a-day schedule. Prescribing smaller, divided daily doses initially helps to avoid accumulation. Prescribing all or most of the longer-acting drugs at bedtime may aid sleep and avoid excessive daytime sedation.

PHARMACOLOGY OF SPECIFIC BENZODIAZEPINES

Chlordiazepoxide

Chlordiazepoxide is the oldest benzodiazepine. It is rapidly and almost completely absorbed after oral administration, but is erratically absorbed after intramuscular (IM) administration. For this reason, IM use of chlordiazepoxide should be avoided. The drug may be given intravenously (IV) if parenteral administration is required. Peak plasma levels occur in 1 to 4 hours after oral administration, and the drug is highly protein-bound. The plasma half-life of chlordiazepoxide ranges from 6 to 30 hours. However, it is transformed into three active metabolites that prolong the activity of the drug. One of these metabolites, desmethyldiazepam, is very long-acting (with an approximate half-life of 48 to 96 hours). Thus, chlordiazepoxide has a tendency to accumulate when it is given several times a day. Patients who are elderly or who have impaired liver function metabolize the drug more slowly and must be watched for the sedative effects of accumulation.

Diazepam

Diazepam is the prototype antianxiety drug. Most clinicians regard it as highly effective, well tolerated, and very safe. It is highly lipid-soluble and water-insoluble, as opposed to chlordiazepoxide, which is water-soluble. Thus, parenteral preparations of diazepam will precipitate if diluted with water or saline. It is rapidly and almost completely absorbed from the gastrointestinal tract. Like chlordiazepoxide, it is erratically and incompletely absorbed after IM administration. However, there is a report that diazepam is well absorbed if injected specifically into the deltoid muscle. When used IV, it should be given slowly (not faster than 10 mg/min) to avoid respiratory depression.

Diazepam is highly protein-bound. Its plasma half-life is between 20 and 50 hours but, like chlordiazepoxide, it is metabolized more slowly by the elderly, in whom the half-life is approximately 90 hours. Diazepam is metabolized into three active metabolites, one of which is desmethyldiazepam. Another metabolite, oxazepam, is marketed as a separate drug. The ratio of diazepam to desmethyldiazepam in the blood is approximately 2:1. Because of its relatively long half-life and its active metabolites, diazepam will accumulate if doses are given too frequently. Special precautions should be taken with its use in the elderly, who are at risk for oversedation and ataxia and their sequelae (falling, hip fractures), and in patients with impaired liver function (especially alcoholics).

Diazepam has become popular as a drug of abuse, most likely because of its rapid absorption, high lipid solubility, and high milligram potency combining to produce acute intoxication. However, there is little evidence that diazepam has significant abuse potential in properly diagnosed and properly treated patients. Its long half-life is an advantage in reducing the likelihood of a withdrawal reaction if the patient inadvertently stops the drug abruptly.

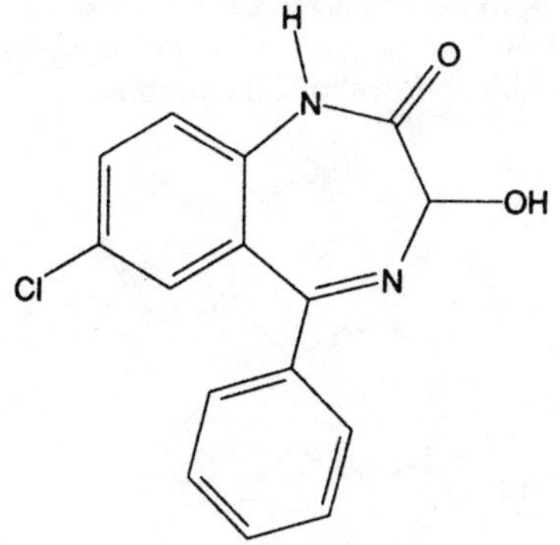

Oxazepam

Oxazepam is one of the metabolites of diazepam. It does not have active metabolites of its own. Oxazepam is conjugated to an inactive glucuronide by the liver and excreted. It has the shortest half-life of any benzodiazepine, approximately 7 hours. Because of its short half-life and lack of any active metabolites, it has little tendency to accumulate with repeated doses. Thus, it may be particularly useful in the geriatric patient or the patient with liver dysfunction. Oxazepam is well absorbed orally and reaches peak plasma levels in 2 to 4 hours. It is highly protein-bound, like chlordiazepoxide and diazepam. Oxazepam is one of the least potent benzodiazepines on a milligram-per-milligram basis and is not available in a parenteral form.

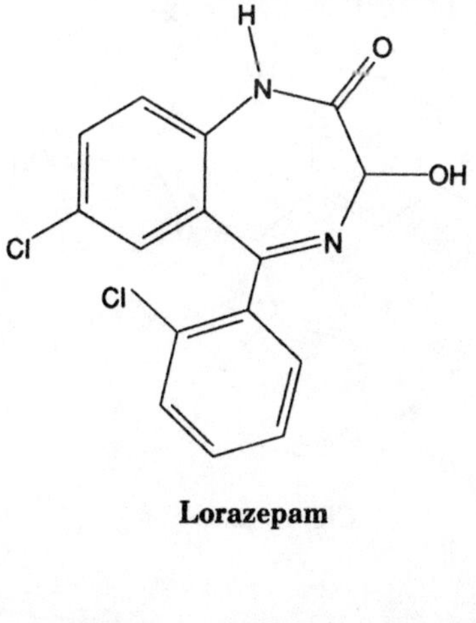

Lorazepam

Lorazepam, like oxazepam, has no active metabolites. Its metabolism is also accomplished by conjugation to an inactive glucuronide. Its plasma half-life is 12 to 15 hours. As with oxazepam, it has less tendency to accumulate than the other benzodiazepines. Peak plasma levels are reached 2 hours after oral administration. Lorazepam is one of the more potent benzodiazepines on a milligram-per-milligram basis, approximately five times the potency of diazepam. It is available in parenteral form and is well-absorbed with given IM (in contrast to chlordiazepoxide and diazepam). The use of IM lorazepam is an effective adjunctive treatment for psychotic agitation in mania and schizophrenia when combined with antipsychotic medication.

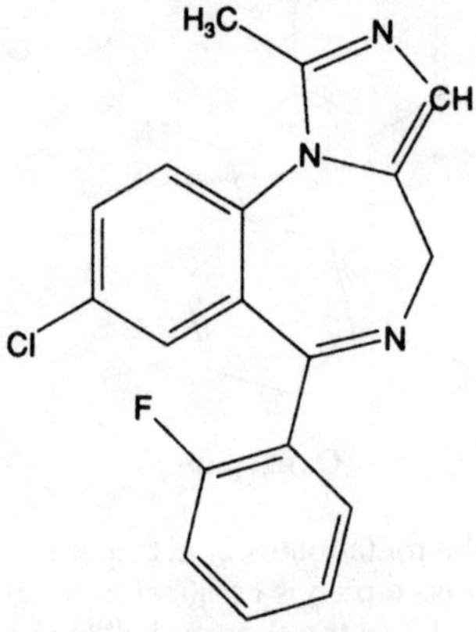

Midazolam

Midazolam is water-soluble and is not painful when injected. It has a more rapid onset of action than diazepam, has a higher milligram-per-milligram potency, and is rapidly eliminated. It is available only in a parenteral form, and is used as an induction agent for anesthesia and for preoperative sedation.

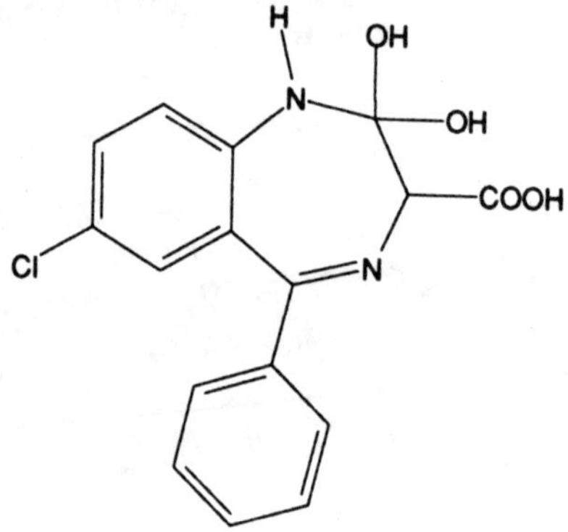

Clorazepate

Clorazepate, itself pharmacologically inactive, is converted in the stomach to desmethyldiazepam, which is the active metabolite of the drug. To accomplish this conversion normal gastric acidity is required. Thus, antacids or achlorhydria will interfere with the efficacy of this agent. The plasma half-life of clorazepate is the same as the half-life of desmethyldiazepam (48 to 96 hours). Because of its long half-life, accumulation can become a problem with this drug. Clorazepate is not available in a parenteral form.

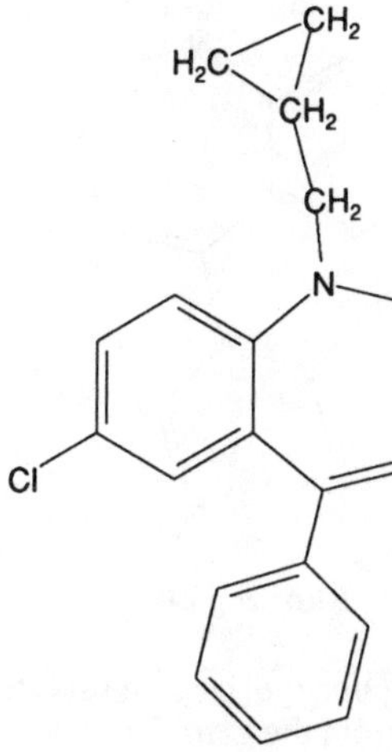

Prazepam

Prazepam is absorbed slowly after oral administration and reaches peak plasma levels of its major metabolite, desmethyldiazepam, in about 6 hours. Its clinical activity is due mainly to desmethyldiazepam. It has a long half-life of approximately 48 to 96 hours, and accumulation of the drug can occur. It is not available in a parenteral form.

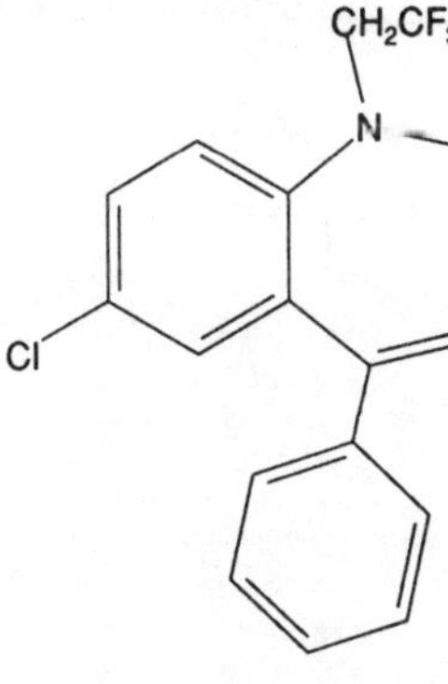

Halazepam

Halazepam is a low potency benzodiazepine whose major active metabolite is also desmethyldiazepam. Its half-life is approximately 14 hours, but it is a long-acting drug due to its conversion to desmethyldiazepam, which has a half-life of 48 to 96 hours. Thus, accumulation can occur with repeated doses. It is not available in a parenteral form.

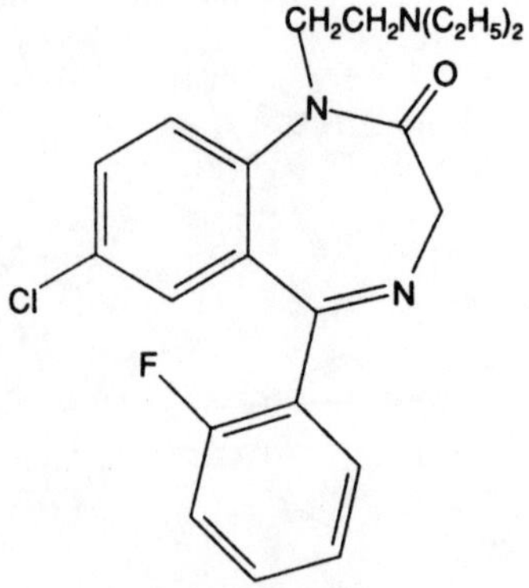

$CH_2CH_2N(C_2H_5)_2$

Flurazepam

Flurazepam is a long-acting benzodiazepine used for the treatment of insomnia. It is rapidly absorbed from the gastrointestinal tract and achieves peak plasma levels in 30 to 60 minutes. Its major active metabolite, N-desalkyl-flurazepam, has a half-life of 47 to 100 hours (longer in the elderly). Thus, accumulation of this metabolite can occur after repeated doses of flurazepam. Clinically, drug hangover is not a frequent problem with flurazepam. In fact, the long half-life may be an advantage for patients with daytime anxiety. However, elderly patients and patients with impaired liver function are at risk for accumulation of this metabolite and should be observed closely.

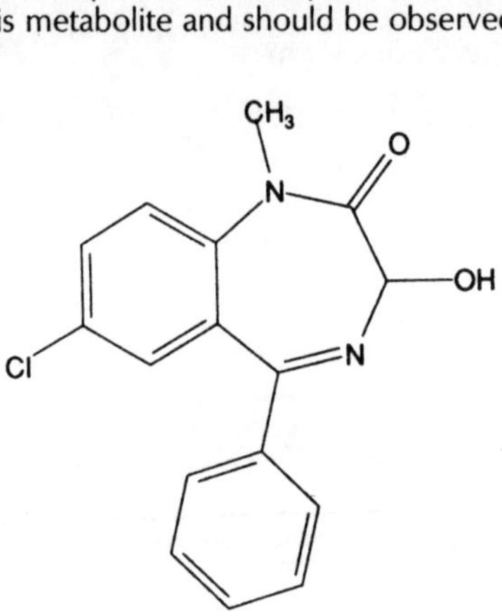

CH_3

Temazepam

Temazepam is also used for insomnia. Absorption is much less rapid than with flurazepam, and it requires 2 to 3 hours to achieve peak plasma levels. It is therefore less useful for patients with sleep-onset insomnia. It has a shorter half-life than flurazepam, about 10 to 15 hours, and has no active metabolites. Because of this, residual daytime sedation is less common. This drug is available in Europe in a soft gel capsule, which promotes more rapid absorption.

Quazepam

Quazepam is a recently released long-acting hypnotic with an elimination half-life of 39 hours. It has two active metabolites with half-lives of 39 and 73 hours, respectively. Its activity will persist into the next day, but to a lesser extent than flurazepam. It is rapidly absorbed from the gastrointestinal tract.

Triazolam

Triazolam is the shortest-acting hypnotic drug, with a half-life of 2 to 5 hours. It is rapidly and well-absorbed after oral administration. Triazolam does not accumulate with repeated use and does not have residual effects on daytime alertness or performance. Unlike flurazepam, however, triazolam will not alleviate daytime anxiety. Because of its short half-life, triazolam is a good choice for elderly patients. However, some clinicians have observed cases in which patients experience a dysphoric withdrawal effect (rebound anxiety) in the morning. Rebound insomnia, a worsening of the sleep disorder after discontinuing the hypnotic, is also more commonly seen with the shorter-acting hypnotics.

Alprazolam

Alprazolam is classified as a triazolobenzodiazepine because of the presence of a fused triazolo ring in the benzodiazepine structure. This difference in structure appears to impart unique properties to alprazolam. In addition to its antianxiety effects, alprazolam also has antidepressant and antipanic activity. It has recently been approved by the Food and Drug Administration for the treatment of panic disorder. It should be thought of as having mild-to-moderate antidepressant effects and is best suited for the treatment of mild-to-moderate depression associated with anxiety. It is not as potent as the tricyclic antidepressants and thus not as effective in the treatment of seriously depressed patients. It is therefore most often used in treating depressed outpatients. Alprazolam does have the advantage of not possessing the cardiovascular and anticholinergic side effects associated with the tricyclic antidepressants. This makes it especially useful for medically ill and elderly depressed patients. The side-effect profile of alprazolam is essentially the same as that for the other benzodiazepines. Oversedation is the most common side effect associated with its use. The half-life of alprazolam is 12 to 15 hours. It is generally prescribed on a tid or a qid regimen. Because of its relatively short half-life, withdrawal reactions from alprazolam can be more serious than those with other benzodiazepines. When discontinuing alprazolam, the drug should be tapered very gradually. The manufacturer recommends tapering the drug no more rapidly than 0.5 mg every 3 days. However, this schedule may be too rapid for most patients, especially those who have been on high doses for a long period of time. A reduction in dose of 0.25 mg every 3 to 7 days appears to be better tolerated by patients clinically. A long-acting preparation (Xanax SR) is currently being investigated. The usual daily dose range of alprazolam for the treatment of anxiety is 0.75 mg to 4 mg/d. Mild to moderately depressed outpatients usually respond to doses between 1.5 mg to 4 mg/d. Doses higher than 4 mg/d may be needed for the treatment of panic disorder. The maximum recommended dose is 10 mg/d.

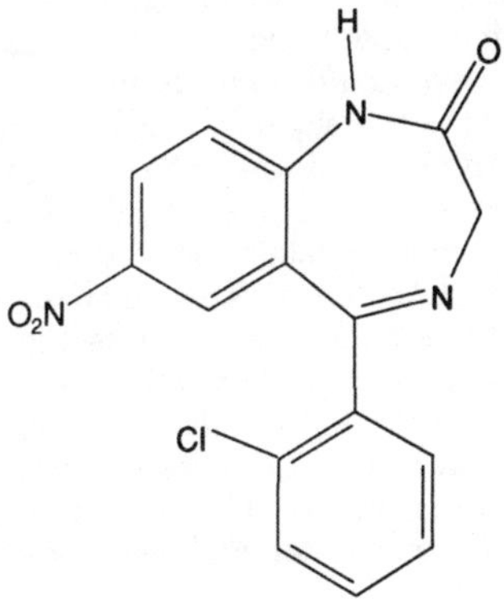

Clonazepam

Clonazepam was initially used for the treatment of akinetic and myoclonic seizures in children. It also appears to have antipanic activity and, as discussed previously, has been used in the treatment of mania. It has the advantage over alprazolam of having a much longer half-life (18 to 42 hours), less likelihood of dependence, and a much lower probability of a withdrawal reaction. A possible disadvantage is that it might cause depression.

OTHER AGENTS USED FOR ANXIETY AND INSOMNIA

Azaspirones

Buspirone represents a new non-benzodiazepine class of antianxiety drugs—the azaspirones (technically, the azaspirodecanediones).

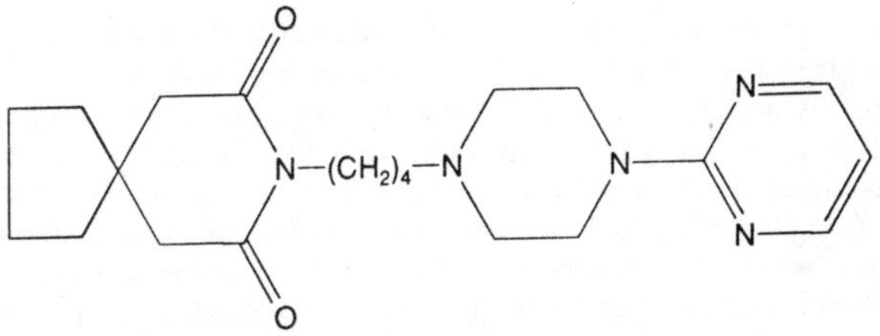

Buspirone

The chemistry and pharmacology of buspirone is unrelated to the benzodiazepines, barbiturates, and other sedative-hypnotic drugs. It does not influence benzodiazepine receptors or GABA. It does not have anticonvulsant, muscle relaxant, or sedative effects and does not appear to present a risk of addiction. It is believed to inhibit the presynaptic serotonin ($5-HT_{1A}$) receptor. Its onset of action resembles the tricyclics, with as long as a 1-month delay after starting treatment. Therefore, it is not appropriate for acute anxiety states. The therapeutic dose range is 20 to 60 mg per day. Most patients may be started on 5 mg tid, with the dose being gradually increased over a month's time. The most commonly reported side effects are nausea, dizziness, headache, and tension. These are generally mild. Buspirone may be particularly useful for the treatment of patients who are addiction-prone (such as alcoholics) or elderly (who may be adversely affected by the sedative side effects of benzodiazepines). The drug must be taken continuously, in contrast to many benzodiazepines that can be taken on an as-needed basis. Our collective clinical experience with buspirone is too short to suggest it as the treatment of choice for any specific anxiety disorder. Buspirone was originally developed as an antipsychotic (having affinity for brain D_2-dopamine receptors). It may also have antidepressant activity. Caution should be exercised because of its theoretical potential for causing tardive dyskinesia, as suggested by its antidopaminergic activity. However, this has not been reported to be a problem clinically.

Beta-Blockers

Beta-blockers are used for the treatment of the autonomic symptoms of anxiety.

Propranolol (Inderal) is the most commonly used beta-blocker in psychiatry.

Propranolol

Beta-blockers compete with norepinephrine and epinephrine at β-adrenergic receptor sites. They have been used since the 1960s for the treatment of anticipatory anxiety (performance anxiety, stage fright). Propranolol, metoprolol, atenolol, and nadolol are used primarily to treat autonomic symptoms such as tachycardia, dry mouth, and tremor. The average dose of propranolol is 10 to 60 mg, usually taken 30 minutes before the anticipated stressor. The main side effects of beta-blockers are bradycardia, hypotension (causing dizziness, light-headedness, and fainting), and excessive sedation. They may also cause depression.

Sedative Antihistamines

Hydroxyzine (Vistaril, Atarax) and diphenhydramine (Benadryl) are two examples of sedative antihistamines.

$$CH_2CH_2OCH_2CH_2OH$$

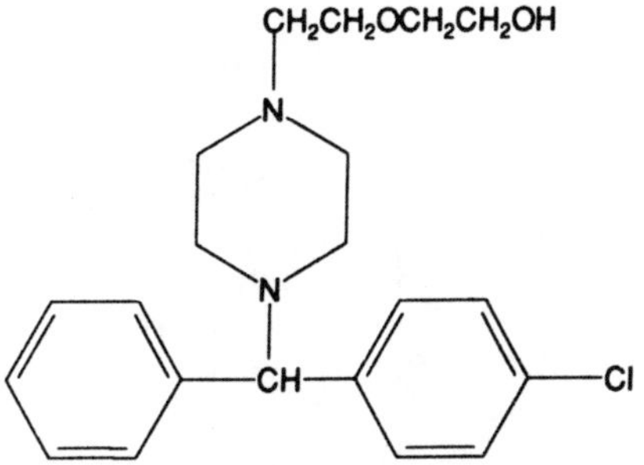

Hydroxyzine

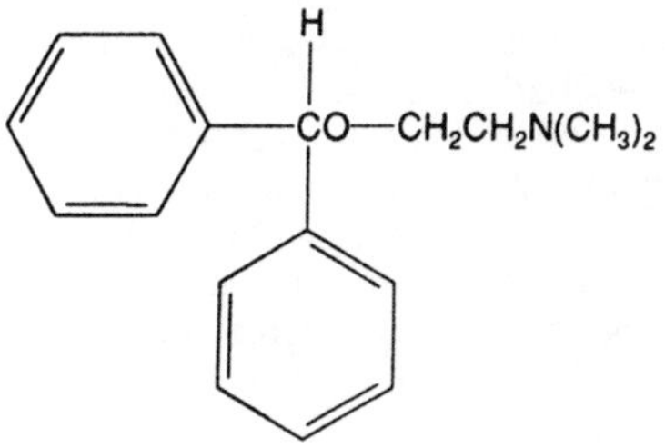

Diphenhydramine

Antihistamines have no muscle-relaxing properties and lower the seizure threshold. Some physicians prescribe these drugs because of their low abuse potential. Because they produce "mental clouding" along with their sedative effect, patients often find them unpleasant compared with the benzodiazepines. However, these drugs may have a special use in the treatment of anxious patients with dermatological disorders (e.g., urticaria, pruritis, neurodermatitis) because of their combined sedative and antihistaminic properties. Hydroxyzine also has antiemetic properties and has been used to treat preoperative nausea and vomiting and motion sickness. These agents have undesirable anticholinergic side effects, and tolerance may develop to their sedative effects. Diphenhydramine has been shown to significantly depress REM sleep in doses of 50 mg. Overall, these agents are not as efficacious in the treatment of anxiety and insomnia as the benzodiazepines. However, they may be useful for patients who have a history of abuse of sedative drugs, anxiety-related skin conditions, and extrapyramidal symptoms (such as patients taking antipsychotic medications).

Barbiturates

Barbiturates can be divided into three categories (long-acting, short-to-intermediate-acting, and ultrashort-acting) according to the duration of their sedative-hypnotic actions.

Barbiturate Structure

Phenobarbital is the prototype of a long-acting barbiturate. Its half-life is 3 to 4 days. About 30% of phenobarbital is excreted by the kidneys. This is in contrast to the shorter-acting barbiturates, which are metabolized almost entirely by the liver. Phenobarbital is also less lipid-soluble and less tightly protein-bound than the shorter-acting barbiturates. Its use as an antianxiety agent is now obsolete, but it is still used as an anticonvulsant. Because a significant amount is excreted by the kidneys, it may be used cautiously in patients with impaired liver function. Phenobarbital is less a drug of abuse than the shorter-acting barbiturates, and its longer duration of action decreases the risk of developing a severe withdrawal reaction upon abrupt discontinuation.

Phenobarbital

The short-to-intermediate-acting barbiturates include pentobarbital, secobarbital, amobarbital, and butabarbital. The latter two are longer acting than the first two. These drugs have been used for the short-term treatment of insomnia, as preanesthetics, and as adjuncts to anesthesia. Pentobarbital (Nembutal) has often been used to withdraw patients addicted to barbiturates and other sedative-hypnotics. The drugs in this group are the ones most frequently abused, especially pentobarbital and secobarbital.

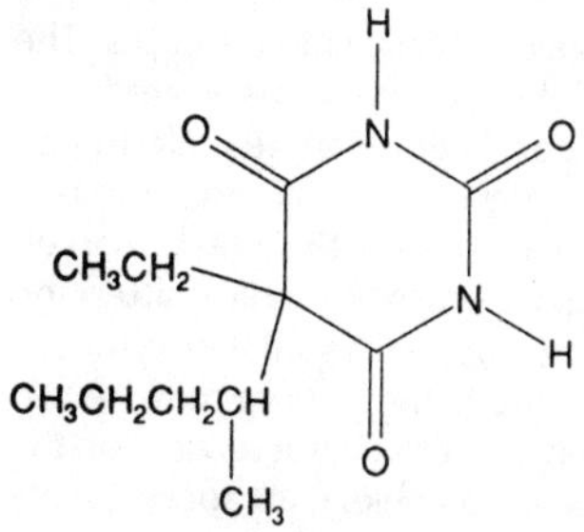

Pentobarbital

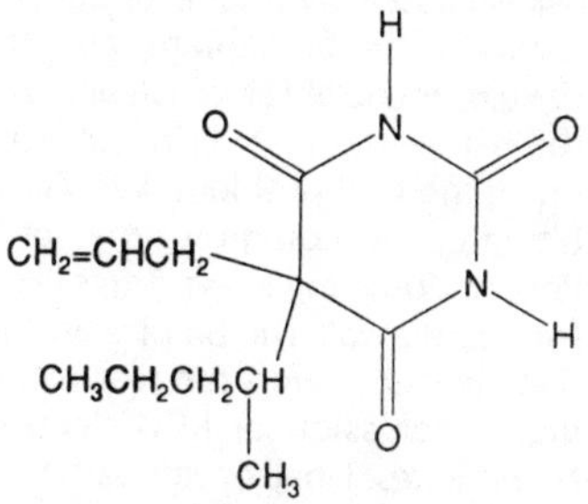

Secobarbital

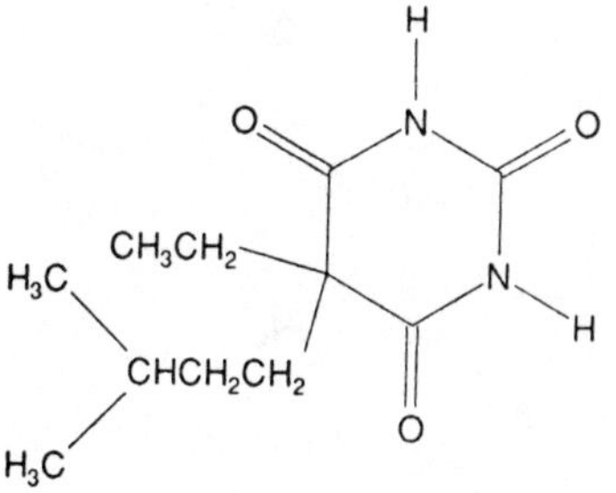

Amobarbital

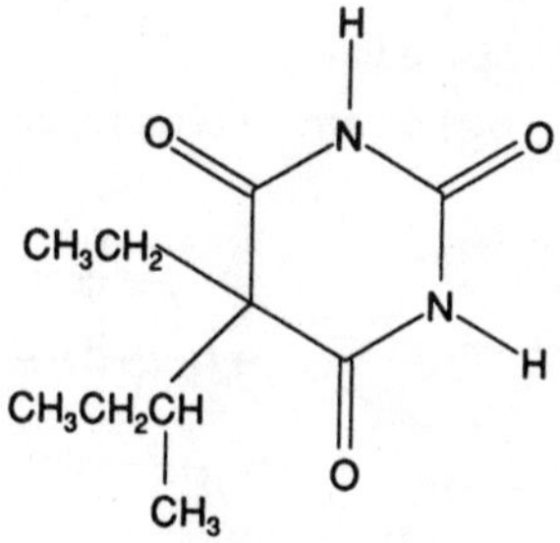

Butabarbital

The ultrashort-acting barbiturates include thiopental and methohexital, which are used intravenously to induce anesthesia.

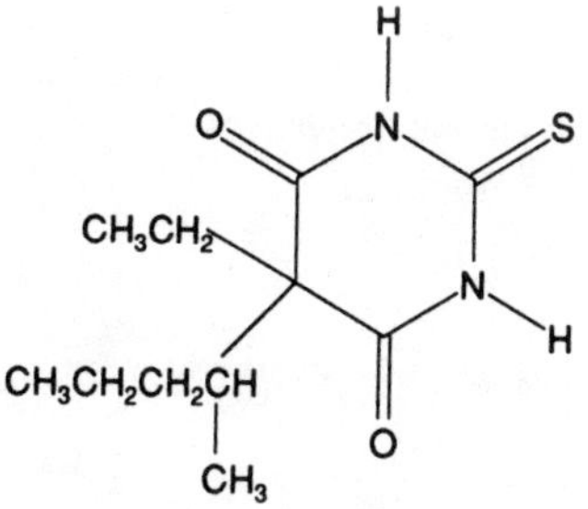

Thiopental

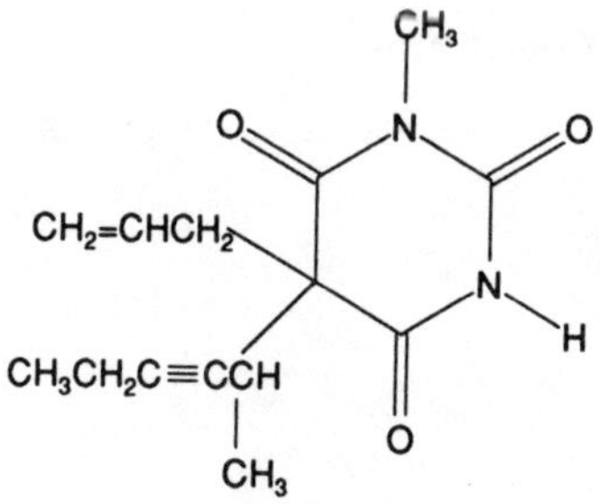

Methohexital

There are several problems with the barbiturates that have led to a decline in their use as antianxiety and hypnotic agents. They have a narrow margin of safety, the lethal dose being relatively close to the therapeutic dose. This risk is caused by their pronounced depressant effect on respiratory centers. Clinically, the barbiturates are often used in successful suicide attempts. The development of tolerance and addiction are other problems associated with the barbiturates. Withdrawal from barbiturate addiction can be a life-threatening medical problem. Withdrawal is complicated by the fact that the barbiturates are common drugs of abuse and available on the black market. People obtaining these drugs illicitly are less likely to seek medical attention for withdrawal. The barbiturates also induce hepatic microsomal enzyme activity, which lowers the plasma levels of other drugs the patient may be taking. Suppression of REM sleep is another unwanted characteristic of the barbiturates. Finally, with barbiturates it is difficult to achieve an adequate antianxiety effect without producing excessive sedation. For all the above reasons, most clinicians now consider the barbiturates to be obsolete for the treatment of anxiety and insomnia.

Propanediol

Meprobamate is a propanediol.

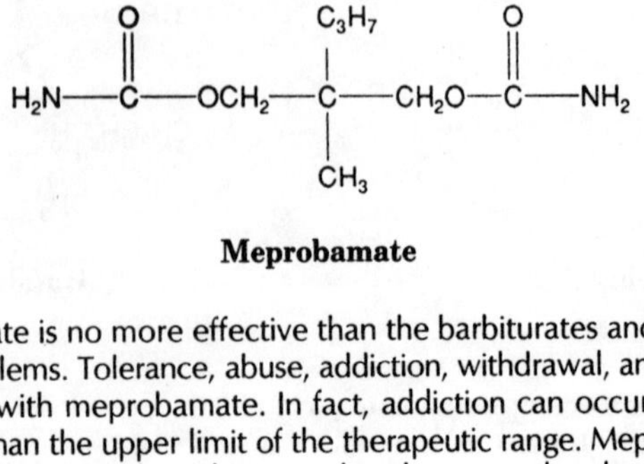

Meprobamate

Meprobamate is no more effective than the barbiturates and has many of the same problems. Tolerance, abuse, addiction, withdrawal, and lethality are all difficulties with meprobamate. In fact, addiction can occur at doses not much higher than the upper limit of the therapeutic range. Meprobamate has a half-life of approximately 12 hours. It does have muscle relaxant properties.

Chloral Derivatives

Chloral hydrate is the principal drug of the chloral derivatives.

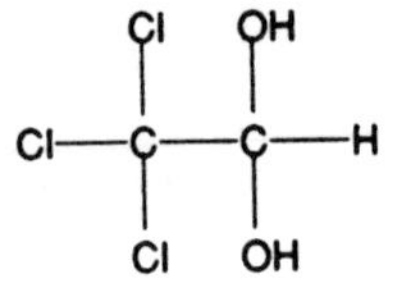

Chloral hydrate

It is metabolized to trichloroacetic acid, which is tightly protein-bound. This characteristic is important clinically because it can displace other drugs that are protein-bound and result in a potentiation of their clinical effect. Chloral hydrate is a relatively safe and rapidly effective hypnotic that appears to be better for sleep induction than sleep maintenance. However, it tends to lose its effectiveness after 1 to 2 weeks of continued use. Its main side effect is gastric irritation. It does not suppress REM sleep or induce hepatic microsomal enzyme activity as much as the barbiturates, and it is also much less abused. Chloral hydrate has a half-life of approximately 8 hours. The usual hypnotic dose is 500 to 1000 mg taken 15 to 30 minutes before bedtime.

Nonbarbiturate Hypnotics

Glutethimide (Doriden), ethchlorvynol (Placidyl), methyprylon (Noludar), and methaqualone (Quaalude) are all non-barbiturate hypnotics (methaqualone has been subsequently taken off the market).

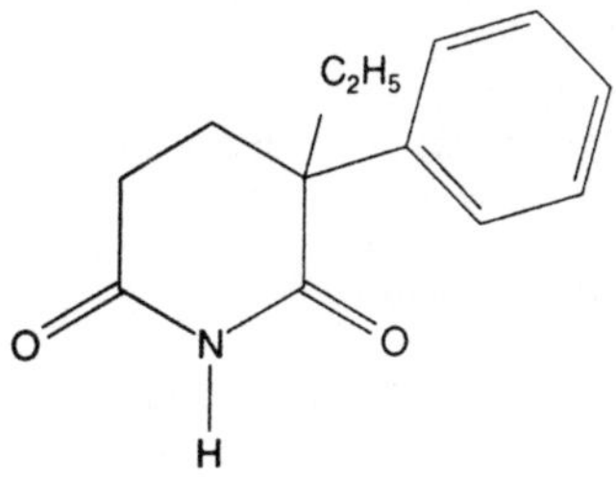

Glutethimide

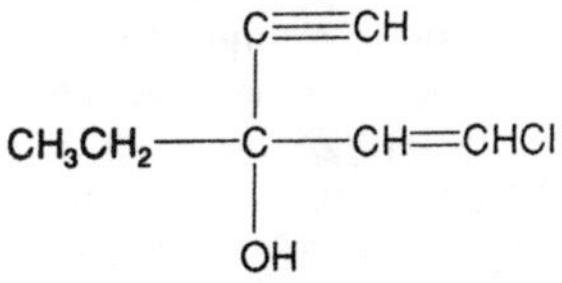

Ethchlorvynol

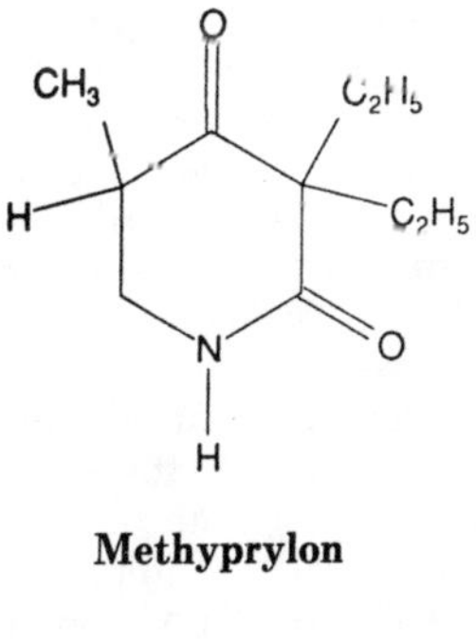

Methyprylon

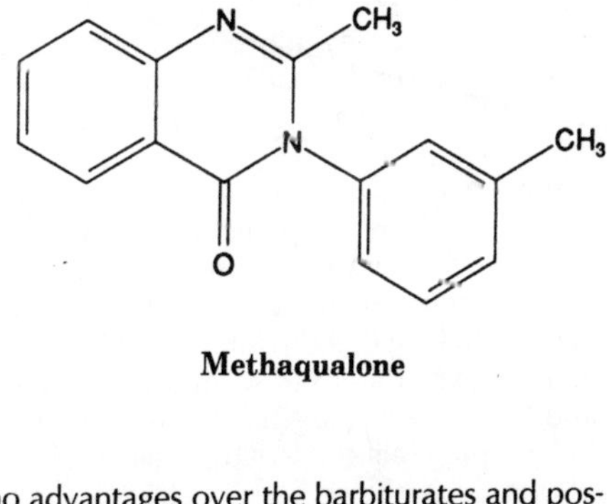

Methaqualone

In general, these drugs have no advantages over the barbiturates and possess many of the same problems. Glutethimide is an extremely lethal drug when taken in overdose. Methaqualone was a popular drug of abuse until it was taken off the market. None of these agents can be recommended for use.

Over-the-Counter Hypnotic Preparations

Over-the-counter drugs are sleeping aids such as Sominex. Although in the past these agents contained harmful drugs (methapyrilene, scopolamine), they now most often contain diphenhydramine (Benadryl). Unisom contains doxylamine succinate, another sedating antihistamine.

INDICATIONS AND GUIDELINES FOR CLINICAL USE

Any patient presenting with a complaint of anxiety could have a medical problem. The most common medical causes of anxiety are cardiovascular, pulmonary, endocrine, and toxic. Myocardial infarction, paroxysmal atrial tachycardia, hypoxia, hypoglycemia, hyperthyroidism, hypoparathyroidism, pheochromocytoma, and caffeine or other drug intoxication are common medical causes of anxiety syndromes. Complaints of anxiety usually present in an outpatient setting where the medical history, review of systems, physical examination, and a battery of screening tests are likely to be less extensive than in the hospital setting. Any patient who is presumed to have a nonmedical psychiatric disorder that does not respond well to psychiatric treatment should have a thorough medical workup.

Once a patient is started on a benzodiazepine, he or she should be followed as frequently as once a week while the dosage is being adjusted and the lowest effective dose is found. The patient may then be seen less often, depending on the need for concurrent psychotherapy and follow-up, from biweekly to monthly. An attempt should be made to determine whether some other type of therapy (e.g., relaxation, marital, family) will help the patient develop a better way of coping with anxiety. How long these drugs are used depends on the individual case. In most cases, patients who are suffering from anxiety caused by temporary stress will require therapy for only a few days or weeks. Long-term treatment is indicated for patients with familial anxiety disorders (who may be presumed to have an inherited disease) and those who are being exposed to unavoidable chronic stress. The best way to determine the need for continued medication is through the trial-and-error approach of gradual dose reduction. The patient may be tapered from the drug and the drug may be successfully discontinued, or the patient may become symptomatic at a lower dose and require continued treatment just above that dose level. Benzodiazepines should always be discontinued gradually to avoid withdrawal symptoms. This practice is especially important with the short- and intermediate-acting drugs such as oxazepam, lorazepam, and alprazolam.

1. *Generalized anxiety disorder* is characterized by the chronic presence of motor tension, autonomic hyperactivity, and hypervigilance. Patients with this disorder complain of such symptoms as nervousness, shakiness, fatigue, difficulty catching their breath, palpitations, sweating, dry mouth, feeling dizzy all the time, stomach discomfort, hot flashes, frequent urination, irritability, and trouble falling asleep. Excessive worrying is the hallmark of the disorder, but it is more difficult to judge objectively than the specific symptomatic complaints.

A standard treatment is diazepam 5 mg tid. Some patients may need less and others as much as 10 mg three or four times a day. The other benzodiazepines are equally efficacious in the treatment of anxiety, and the choice of drug should be based on the patient's individual needs. The longer-acting

ANTIANXIETY DRUGS 111

benzodiazepines are prone to accumulate and cause oversedation, while the shorter-acting drugs have been associated with withdrawal reactions upon abrupt discontinuation. Usual daily dose ranges for the benzodiazepines are listed in Table 4.1.

Although it is hard to prove, it is the impression of many clinicians that generalized anxiety disorder runs in families. It is also observed to follow episodes of major depression. The consequences of failing to treat it may include alcoholism, progression to a major depression, and suicide.

It would hardly be possible to help an anxious patient without having a psychotherapeutic relationship. Perhaps the most difficult part of the psychotherapy is persuading the patient to take medication in the first place, particularly because of the current state of psychopharmacologic politics. The patient needs to be informed that benzodiazepine drugs, taken in therapeutic doses, do not lead to addiction of the kind portrayed in the media and should not be compared to hard drugs.

Like any other medication, a benzodiazepine should be prescribed for a specifically diagnosed disorder along with the appropriate nonbiological treatments (psychological and social therapies), reassessed periodically during continued use, avoided in high-risk patients, titrated to achieve the best possible balance between efficacy and side effects, monitored for abuse, tapered to the lowest effective dose, and reevaluated with respect to the accuracy of the original diagnosis. Although it is unlikely to be physiologically harmful to continue the patient on a fixed dose of a benzodiazepine, it is good medical practice to continue to seek the lowest effective dose, while offering psychotherapy to help the patient learn to cope better with stress and provide him or her

Table 4.1. Benzodiazepines

GENERIC NAME	TRADE NAME	SPEED OF ONSET	DURATION OF ACTION	USUAL DAILY DOSE RANGE (mg/d)*
Antianxiety drugs				
Alprazolam†	Xanax	Rapid	Intermediate	0.75–4
Chlordiazepoxide†	Librium	Intermediate	Long	15–100
Clonazepam	Klonopin	Intermediate	Long	0.75–4
Clorazepate‡	Tranxene	Rapid	Long	15–60
Diazepam‡	Valium	Rapid	Long	4–40
Halazepam	Paxipam	Slow	Long	40–160
Lorazepam‡	Ativan	Intermediate	Intermediate	1–6
Oxazepam‡	Serax	Slow	Short	30–120
Prazepam‡	Centrax	Slow	Long	20–60
Hypnotic drugs				
Flurazepam‡	Dalmane	Rapid	Long	15–30
Quazepam	Doral	Rapid	Long	7.5–15
Temazepam‡	Restoril	Slow	Intermediate	15–30
Triazolam	Halcion	Rapid	Short	0.125–0.25

*Higher doses may be needed for the treatment of alcohol withdrawal.
†Higher doses may be needed for the treatment of panic disorder.
‡Also available generically.

with more permanent ways of dealing with anxiety. Psychotherapy alone, however, is often not effective in the treatment of generalized anxiety disorder. Because of its chronicity, generalized anxiety disorder should, at least on theoretical grounds, respond well to buspirone, but the comparative efficacy of buspirone in this disorder is yet to be established.

2. *Adjustment disorder with anxious mood.* Patients with situational anxiety have just undergone an emotionally traumatic experience (marital separation, rape, serious auto accident, presence of a medical illness) and are candidates for brief crisis-intervention psychotherapy combined with benzodiazepine therapy. In uncomplicated cases diazepam 5 mg tid or lorazepam 1 mg tid are average doses. Benzodiazepines may be needed acutely for overwhelming anxiety, as well as for the insomnia that follows. Proper treatment of adjustment disorders with combined psychotherapy and pharmacotherapy has the potential for preventing the development of posttraumatic stress disorder and pathological grief reactions.

3. *Panic disorder* can be treated with antidepressant drugs. It also responds to alprazolam. This triazolobenzodiazepine drug has combined antidepressant–antianxiety activity and is one of the drugs of choice for panic disorder. The therapeutic range for alprazolam in panic disorder is generally 2 to 6 mg daily in divided doses. The anticonvulsant–antianxiety drug clonazepam has also been used effectively to treat panic disorder. Whether to use a tricyclic antidepressant or alprazolam or clonazepam depends on several factors involving differences in efficacy, side effects, and risk of dependence.

The conventional benzodiazepines are useful in the treatment of anticipatory anxiety in patients with agoraphobia and for patients facing anxiety-provoking situations, although the latter might be considered for treatment with beta-blockers.

An important aspect of the management of all anxiety disorders is the degree to which the problem can be understood and treated as biological (genetically inherited, caused by a medical disease), psychological (psychodynamically meaningful, the result of learning), or social (resulting from stress, lack of social support). Often a combination of such factors needs to be taken into account in order to formulate the case. The patient may require a benzodiazepine combined with psychosocial therapies aimed specifically at points where the greatest leverage for alleviation of impaired function can be obtained.

4. *Social phobia* is characterized by fear of being scrutinized in public. Social phobia ranges from stage fright to fear of saying foolish things in social situations. Anxiety symptoms are typically peripheral (noradrenergic) rather than central (GABAergic) and may respond more specifically to a beta-blocker like propranolol than to a benzodiazepine. Another advantage of using a beta-blocker for such patients is that it is more likely to preserve normal adaptive alertness in social situations. Monoamine oxidase inhibitors are also used for social phobia.

5. *Simple phobia* is a circumscribed fear that produces an immediate anxiety response in confrontation with the feared object (typically animals, closed spaces, heights, and air travel). The patient may avoid the phobic object in order to prevent anticipatory anxiety. Behavior therapy is the best treatment for simple phobia, but it can take a long time. If the patient needs immediate help (e.g., must travel on an airplane), the prescription of diazepam, 5 to 10 mg,

or lorazepam, 1 to 2 mg, is advised. Interestingly, possession of the prescribed medication alone may provide reassurance and reduce phobic anxiety to the point where the medication is not actually taken.

6. *Obsessive compulsive disorder.* The presence of obsessions or compulsions defines this disorder. Benzodiazepines play a limited role in the treatment of this disorder, although high-dose alprazolam has been reported to cause symptomatic improvement. The drugs of choice are the specifically antiobsessional antidepressants, clomipramine and fluoxetine.

7. *Major depression.* Benzodiazepines play a limited role in the treatment of mood disorders. Although not a drug of choice, alprazolam is useful for the treatment of depression in patients who cannot tolerate conventional antidepressants. These include patients who are intolerant to anticholinergic and hypotensive effects as well as medically ill patients with cardiovascular problems and elderly patients for whom a hypotensive episode, anticholinergic delirium, or arrhythmia could be disastrous. In the opinion of some clinicians, alprazolam has high specificity and efficacy for recently precipitated anxious depressions of mild-to-moderate severity and has a rapid response time. Therefore, it may reduce both morbidity and mortality in a subgroup of major depressives.

Depression accompanied by anxiety may respond better to monoamine oxidase inhibitors than tricyclic antidepressants, but the anxiety the average patient feels when informed about the risk of a hypertensive crisis is enough to eliminate the advantage in many cases. The use of benzodiazepines during the first week or two of tricyclic antidepressant therapy can reduce anxiety and lessen or eliminate insomnia, which is often the most painful aspect of major depression. Alprazolam, 0.5 to 1 mg tid or qid, is a good choice for adjunctive treatment of anxiety with a tricyclic antidepressant. It has the advantage of having antidepressant activity itself, and is therefore unlikely to worsen the patient's depression. Flurazepam, 30 mg hs, is helpful for patients with severe insomnia associated with depression. Triazolam, 0.125 to 0.25 mg hs, may also be helpful. Antipsychotics can be effectively used for agitated and delusional depressives.

8. *Alcohol withdrawal and alcohol withdrawal delirium* are best treated with benzodiazepines because of their greater safety and efficacy compared with the other cross-tolerant drugs. Tremulousness and elevations of blood pressure in the absence of delirium can often be treated with doses of diazepam ranging from 5 to 10 mg q4h prn. The medication is then tapered over the course of 2 weeks or more. Elderly patients and patients with cirrhosis (impaired liver function) should be treated with oxazepam, 10 to 30 mg, q4h prn, with the same tapering of dose as noted above.

Delirium tremens, associated with hypertension and fever, is a life-threatening medical emergency with a 20% mortality rate and should be treated in an intensive care unit with IV diazepam, 5 to 10 mg q2h prn or lorazepam, 1 to 2 mg q2h prn. Ideal treatment conditions with special attention to medical complications, such as pneumonia and subdural hematoma, have reduced the mortality rate in some hospitals to 5%.

9. *Psychological factors affecting physical condition.* The benzodiazepines are safe drugs to use for anxiety caused by or contributing to medical disorders, for example, in patients recovering from myocardial infarction. They are also useful in the management of medical problems that are characteristically

associated with anxiety, notably peptic ulcer disease, colitis, and irritable bowel syndrome. Benzodiazepines are not the only psychotropic drugs useful for the management of these types of "psychosomatic" diseases. For example, the highly anticholinergic tricyclic antidepressants doxepin and amitriptyline have been effective in the management of irritable bowel syndrome.

10. *Psychotic disorders* are an indication for the use of benzodiazepines under special circumstances. Benzodiazepines are used as an adjunct or alternative to antipsychotics for the treatment of agitation in mania and schizophrenia. They have been reported to have therapeutic effects on residual symptoms of schizophrenia, specifically social anxiety and negative symptoms. Benzodiazepines have been reported to be dramatically effective in catatonia, although no double-blind studies have been done.

An advantage of benzodiazepines is their short duration of action relative to antipsychotics and the avoidance of extrapyramidal and anticholinergic side effects. Lorazepam is the preferred drug for agitation because of its short half-life and its availability and absorbability in IM form. Lorazepam is typically prescribed in 1 to 2 mg doses IM q1h to q2h prn for acute psychotic agitation. Lorazepam and diazepam have been reported to be effective in catatonia when given IM or IV. Lorazepam and clonazepam have been reported to be effective in the treatment of acute mania.

The most interesting use of benzodiazepines in psychosis suggests that at high doses they have antipsychotic activity. The prescription of 200 to 400 mg of diazepam daily to schizophrenics has been reported to lead to a significant improvement in psychotic symptoms. The mechanism of action is unknown, but it has been suggested that the capacity of benzodiazepines to enhance the activity of the inhibitory neurotransmitter GABA may result in the inhibition of dopamine. This use of benzodiazepines should be considered experimental.

11. *Akathisia* is a common side effect of antipsychotic treatment characterized by restlessness, pacing, and irritability. It may be mistaken for a worsening of the psychosis. This neurologic syndrome responds unpredictably to a variety of drugs: anticholinergics, antihistaminics, clonidine, beta-blockers, and benzodiazepines. The benzodiazepines diazepam (average dose, 5 mg tid) and lorazepam (average dose, 1 mg tid) may be effective in some patients.

12. *Drug-induced psychoses.* These conditions, secondary to illicit hallucinogenic drugs such as lysergic acid diethylamide (LSD), phencyclidine (PCP), mescaline, tetrahydrocannabinol (THC), and others, are an indication for the benzodiazepines if pharmacologic intervention is necessary. Some severe drug-induced psychoses (such as those seen with PCP) may require treatment with an antipsychotic drug. However, many illicit drug preparations contain belladonna alkaloids. The anticholinergic effects of the antipsychotics would tend to potentiate those of the belladonna alkaloids and exacerbate the condition. The benzodiazepines, lorazepam and diazepam, are most often used for this indication. If an antipsychotic drug is required, one with minimal anticholinergic effects (e.g., haloperidol) is recommended.

13. *Nonpsychiatric uses* of benzodiazepines are for anesthetic, preanesthetic and preoperative, anticonvulsant, and muscle-relaxant actions. Diazepam is the drug of choice for status epilepticus, for which it is given intravenously. Although a danger of respiratory depression is present, the risk is less than with phenobarbital. Clonazepam is used for akinetic, myoclonic, and petit mal

seizures. Diazepam is an effective muscle relaxant for patients with trismus (teeth clenching), back strain, and spasticity secondary to cerebral palsy. It has also been used as an adjunctive treatment in tetanus. Diazepam and lorazepam are used IV as short-acting anesthetics prior to cardioversion and other procedures (e.g., bronchoscopy, gastroscopy). When given IV, they tend to produce amnesia for the procedure. Benzodiazepines are also used to reduce preoperative anxiety.

BENZODIAZEPINE TREATMENT OF INSOMNIA

Insomnia is a common problem affecting 15% of the population. It is associated with many different medical and psychiatric conditions. Specific sleep disorders such as sleep apnea syndrome can actually be made worse with benzodiazepines. Certain medical conditions causing insomnia, such as congestive heart failure, should obviously be treated medically, rather than with benzodiazepines. One of the most common psychiatric causes of insomnia is depression, which should be treated with antidepressant medication. There is, however, a residual category of patients who have insomnia for which benzodiazepine treatment is indicated. We now know enough about insomnia to have developed a psychiatric classification that includes the dyssomnias and parasomnias. In the dyssomnias there is a disturbance in the length, quality, or timing of sleep. In the parasomnias a behavioral disturbance occurs during sleep. Primary insomnia is a sleep disorder independent of any known medical or psychiatric condition. Insomnia disorders are dyssomnias characterized by difficulty falling or staying asleep.

1. *Insomnia related to another mental disorder (nonorganic)* may be caused by such illnesses as major depression, generalized anxiety disorder, dementia, schizophrenia, bipolar disorder, posttraumatic stress disorder, adjustment disorder with anxious mood, and personality disorders. Benzodiazepines may be prescribed along with other psychiatric drugs and combined with psychological or social therapies. The use of caffeine and alcohol should be avoided. Flurazepam (Dalmane) 30 mg hs, temazepam (Restoril) 30 mg hs, or triazolam (Halcion) 0.25 mg hs are effective drugs for short-term treatment. Patients who are experiencing continuing reversible stress (grief, stress at work, marital separation) may require treatment for weeks instead of days. There is another group of patients who have persistent insomnia. Although there may have been a precipitating event, they may not have been able to return to a normal sleep pattern. A combination of education, support, sleep schedules, using the bed only for sleep, and reduction of total time in bed may be useful, along with a slow tapering-off of the benzodiazepine, to terminate insomnias that have been conditioned.

2. *Insomnia related to a known organic factor* may be caused by a medical illness or a psychoactive substance use disorder. Physical illnesses commonly cause insomnia by producing pain or discomfort (arthritis, congestive heart failure, nocturia). Medical treatment with certain drugs (amphetamines, bronchodilators, steroids) and psychoactive substance use disorders (e.g., alcohol or amphetamine dependence) can cause insomnia. Sometimes more effective treatment of the medical problem will eliminate the insomnia. At other times, periodic use of a benzodiazepine is helpful. Although dependence on benzodiazepines is preferable to dependence on such drugs as am-

phetamines or alcohol, failure to deal with the primary psychiatric problem of psychoactive substance use could lead, by addition of a benzodiazepine, to irrational polypharmacy or polysubstance abuse.

3. *Primary insomnia* is a residual category of dyssomnias for which no medical or psychiatric cause has been discovered. It should probably be treated behaviorally, with attention to developing a sleep schedule, using the bed only for sleeping, and restricting the time in bed. However, some patients will not improve without benzodiazepine treatment. A low dose of a sedating tricyclic antidepressant may also be tried. If a benzodiazepine is effective, an attempt should be made to slowly taper it to the point of discontinuation. If that is not possible, the patient should be instructed to try taking the benzodiazepine on alternate days, and then to try taking it less frequently until it is only used occasionally on an as-needed basis.

4. *Sleep–wake schedule disorder* may be caused by time-zone changes (jet lag), staying up all night for several days, or a change in work shift. Any delay or advance in onset or offset of sleep can cause this problem. An acute problem like jet lag can usually be treated in a few days with a hypnotic benzodiazepine. Patients who must persist at a new shift generally adapt after a week or so of sleep disruption, which may present with an exacerbation of an underlying psychiatric disorder (e.g., increased anxiety in a patient with panic disorder). A specific behavioral treatment known as chronotherapy has been developed for sleep–wake schedule disorders. This treatment is thought to reset the biological clock by imposing 26 to 27-hour days until normal sleep returns.

5. *Sleep terror disorder* is a parasomnia, characterized by episodes of repeated awakening associated with panicky screams. It usually occurs during non-REM sleep (stages 3 and 4) during the first third of the night. It can often be treated with a benzodiazepine (e.g., diazepam) or a tricyclic antidepressant (e.g., imipramine).

6. *Sleepwalking disorder* is another type of parasomnia in which the patient leaves the bed while asleep, usually during non-REM sleep (sleep stages 3 and 4) during the first third of the night. It can often be treated with a benzodiazepine (e.g., diazepam) or a tricyclic antidepressant (e.g., imipramine).

SIDE EFFECTS

1. The main side effect associated with the use of benzodiazepines is drowsiness. Fatigue, poor concentration, ataxia, dysarthria, and confusion may also occur. In elderly patients, falls and hip fracture have resulted from oversedation with these drugs, prompting the suggestion that buspirone be considered as a safer alternative. Patients should be cautioned about driving, operating heavy machinery, and using alcohol in combination with benzodiazepines. Respiratory depression may occur in patients with preexisting respiratory disease. These agents should not be used in patients with respiratory failure.

2. Occasional patients report feeling irritable, angry, or agitated after having taken benzodiazepines. More rarely, rage reactions have been reported. These have been explained as due to the disinhibiting effect of these agents, similar to that seen with alcohol.

3. Other side effects reported with the benzodiazepines include gastrointestinal discomfort, vertigo, decreased libido, and allergic skin reactions.

4. Tolerance and dependence may develop slowly with the benzodiazepines.

However, a more important clinical problem is psychological dependence (habituation), which may impede the rational reduction and discontinuation of the drug. This is a special problem that tests the psychological resources of the patient and the psychiatrist's knowledge of the psychology and psychopharmacology of anxiety. A relevant aspect of the doctor–patient relationship is that medication may be viewed as a transitional object representing the physician.

5. Benzodiazepines can precipitate or aggravate depression. Some depressions present with anxiety as the chief complaint and pose a problem in diagnosis and treatment. These depressions in particular may be aggravated by benzodiazepine treatment. There is an important exception, however. Alprazolam has a unique antianxiety–antidepressant spectrum of activity and may be the drug of choice for many anxious depressions. It is a matter of clinical judgment whether a patient is more likely to respond well to alprazolam or to a tricyclic antidepressant. In general, patients with unprecipitated depressions who have a full depressive syndrome and little or no anxiety should be started on a tricyclic antidepressant. Patients with severe depressions and agitation (pacing, hand-wringing) should be placed on a tricyclic antidepressant combined with an antipsychotic drug.

6. The serious problems of tolerance and dependence with the barbiturates and meprobamate have been noted before. These drugs also produce side effects because they cause significant depression of the central nervous system. Respiratory depression caused by barbiturates is worse than that produced by benzodiazepines. The barbiturates can produce paradoxical excitement, particularly in the elderly. They may also precipitate or exacerbate acute intermittent porphyria and should not be used in patients with this condition.

USE IN PREGNANCY AND LACTATION

It is no longer thought that the benzodiazepines cause cleft palate abnormalities, but no research has been done to determine that benzodiazepines are safe during pregnancy. It would be prudent to avoid benzodiazepines during pregnancy, especially during the first trimester. Benzodiazepines are excreted in breast milk, and it is advisable that mothers taking benzodiazepines not breast-feed their infants.

USE IN THE ELDERLY

Use short-acting benzodiazepines such as oxazepam, lorazepam, and alprazolam in low doses and increase the dose slowly to avoid excessive accumulation and sedation. The use of longer-acting drugs is likely to lead to oversedation, incoordination, confusion, and consequent risk of hip fracture secondary to falls. The hypnotic triazolam (in a dose of 0.125 mg) is recommended for use in the elderly because of its short half-life.

DRUG INTERACTIONS

1. The sedative effects of the antianxiety and hypnotic drugs will be potentiated by other drugs that also depress the central nervous system. These drugs include tricyclic antidepressants, narcotic analgesics, antipsychotic

agents, antihistamines, and alcohol. The interaction with alcohol is especially important because alcohol is commonly used and abused. Although the benzodiazepines are rarely lethal when taken in overdose, they are much more likely to be lethal when combined with alcohol. Triazolam may be the exception to the rule, as deaths have been reported when this agent has been taken alone in overdose.

2. The barbiturates and glutethimide induce hepatic microsomal enzymes and thus increase the metabolism of other drugs. This process results in decreased blood levels and decreased therapeutic effectiveness. Drugs affected by enzyme induction include the coumarin anticoagulants, tricyclic antidepressants, chlorpromazine, phenytoin, phenylbutazone, corticosteroids, tolbutamide, digitoxin, and vitamin D. Drug interaction with coumarin anticoagulants (Warfarin) can be especially troublesome. Anticoagulant blood levels may rise sharply upon the discontinuation of these enzyme-inducing drugs, resulting in uncontrolled bleeding. Ethchlorvynol may also induce hepatic microsomal enzymes and reduce the blood levels of the oral anticoagulants. Chloral hydrate has been reported to have two different effects on the oral anticoagulants. Enzyme induction similar to that seen with the barbiturates, glutethimide, and ethchlorvynol has been noted. Chloral hydrate also potentiates the effects of the anticoagulants by displacing them from protein-binding sites. The potentiation is a short-term effect, unlike the enzyme induction. Chloral hydrate has also been reported to lower serum levels of tricyclic antidepressants.

3. Benzodiazepines do not induce hepatic microsomal enzymes or produce protein-binding displacement. They produce fewer drug interactions, in general, than any other class of antianxiety or hypnotic drug. They may be used safely with the oral anticoagulants and tricyclic antidepressants.

4. Normal stomach acidity is needed for the breakdown of clorazepate and for the prompt absorption of other benzodiazepines. Antacids interfere with the conversion of clorazepate to desmethyldiazepam in the stomach and therefore decrease the effectiveness of this drug. Antacids have also been reported to delay absorption of other benzodiazepines. Thus, antacids should be avoided with clorazepate and given two hours before or after other benzodiazepines.

5. Disulfiram (Antabuse) has been reported to interfere with the metabolism of chlordiazepoxide and diazepam. Apparently it impedes the demethylation of these drugs, thus reducing their clearance. If a patient is taking disulfiram, one of the benzodiazepines that does not undergo demethylation (e.g., oxazepam, lorazepam) should be used.

6. Benzodiazepines may potentiate the side effects of phenytoin (Dilantin) and in some patients cause toxicity. Impaired coordination, ataxia, drowsiness, restlessness, and irritability may be seen in patients taking this drug combination. Epileptic and other patients taking phenytoin should be observed closely for signs of toxicity resulting from the co-prescription of a benzodiazepine.

7. Cimetidine (Tagamet) has been reported to inhibit the metabolism of diazepam and chlordiazepoxide by the liver, resulting in increased blood levels of these benzodiazepines. This may not be clinically significant but warrants attention. Clorazepate and prazepam are similarly affected. However, cimetidine does not appear to affect the metabolism of oxazepam or lorazepam because these drugs are not as extensively metabolized by the liver.

Bibliography

American Medical Association. AMA drug evaluations. 6th ed. Chicago: American Medical Association; 1986.

Appleton WS. Practical clinical pharmacology. Baltimore, MD: William & Wilkins; 1988.

Barchas JD, Berger PA, Ciaranello RD, Elliott GR (eds). Psychopharmacology from theory to practice. New York: Oxford University Press; 1977.

Baldessarini RJ. Chemotherapy in psychiatry. Cambridge, MA: Harvard University Press; 1985.

Baughman OL. Diagnosis and management of anxiety in the older patient: the role of azaspirones. Advances in Therapy. 1989;6:6, 269–286.

Belmaker RH, VanPraag HM, eds. Mania: an evolving concept. Jamaica, NY: Spectrum; 1980.

Bernstein JG. Drug therapy in psychiatry. Littleton, MA: PSG Publishing Company; 1988.

Cade JFJ. The story of lithium. In Ayd F, Blackwell B, eds. Biological psychiatry. Philadelphia: Lippincott; 1970: 218–229.

Easton MS, Janicak PG. The use of benzodiazepines in psychotic disorders. Psychiatric Annals. 1990;20:535–544.

Eison MS. The new generation of serotonergic anxiolytics. Psychopathology. 1989; 22(suppl 1):13–20.

Ellicott A, Hammen C, Gitlin M, Brown G, Janison K. Life events and the course of bipolar disorder. Am J Psychiatry. 1990;147:1194–1198.

Elkes J. Discoveries in biological psychiatry. New York: Lippincott; 1970.

Gilman AG, Rall TW, Nies AS, Taylor P. Goodman and Gilman's The Pharmacologic basis of therapeutics. 8th ed. Elmsford, NY: Pergamon Press; 1990.

Goodwin FK, Jamison KR. Manic-Depressive Illness. New York: Oxford University Press; 1990.

Guttmacher LB. Concise guide to somatic therapies in psychiatry. Washington, DC: American Psychiatric Press; 1988.

Hollister LE. Clinical pharmacology of psychotherapeutic drugs. 3rd ed. New York: Churchill Livingstone; 1990.

Hollister LE, ed. Psychopharmacology: drug side-effects and interactions. In Hales RE, Frances AJ, eds. American Psychiatric Association annual review. Vol. 6, Washington, DC: American Psychiatric Association Press; 1987; 698–821.

Hyman SE, Arana GW. Handbook of psychiatric drug therapy. Boston: Little Brown; 1987.

Janowsky DS, Addario D, Risch SC. Psychopharmacology case studies. New York: Guilford; 1987.

Jefferson JW. Lithium: the present and the future. J. Clin Psychiatry. 1990;51(8,suppl):4–8.

Jefferson JW, Greist JH, Ackerman DL, Carroll JA. Lithium encyclopedia for clinical practice. Washington, DC: American Psychiatric Press; 1987.

Johnson J, Weismann MM, Klerman GL. Panic disorder, comorbidity, and suicide attempts. Arch Gen Psychiatry. 1990;47:805–808.

Klein DF, Gittelman R, Quitkin F, Rifkin A. Diagnosis and drug treatment of psychiatric disorders. Baltimore: William & Wilkins; 1980.

Lazare A, ed. Outpatient psychiatry. Baltimore: William & Wilkins; 1989.

Levitt AJ, Joffe RT, Ennis J, MacDonald C, Kutcher SP. The prevalence of cyclothymia in borderline personality disorder. J Clin Psychiatry. 1990;51:335–339.

Lion JR. The art of medicating psychiatric patients. Baltimore: William & Wilkins; 1978.

Mason AS, Granacher RP. Clinical handbook of antipsychotic drug therapy. New York: Brunner/Mazel; 1980.

Meltzer HY, ed. Psychopharmacology: the third generation of progress. New York: Raven Press; 1987.

Nemeroff CB. Use and abuse of benzodiazepines. Audio-Digest Psychiatry. 1990;19:12.

Nicholi AM, ed. The new Harvard guide to modern psychiatry. Cambridge, MA: Harvard University Press; 1988.

Oken D, Lacovics M, (eds). A clinical manual of psychiatry. New York: Elsevier/North-Holland; 1982.

Paul SM. Anxiety and depression: a common neurobiological substrate? J Clin Psychiatry. 1988;49(10, suppl):13–16.

Pirodsky DM. Primer of clinical psychopharmacology: a practical guide. Garden City, NY: Medical Examination Publishing Co.; 1981.

Post RM, Trimble MR, Pippenger CD. Clinical use of anticonvulsants in psychiatric disorders. New York: Demos; 1989.

Ray WA, Griffin MR, Schaffner W, Baugh DK, Melton LJ III. Psychotropic drug use and risk of hip fracture. N Engl J Med. 1987;316:363.

Rifkin A, Doddi S, Karajgi B, Hasan N, Alvarez L. Benzodiazepine use and abuse at outpatient clinics. Am J Psychiatry. 1989;146:1331.

Rizack MA, Hillman CDM. The medical letter handbook of adverse drug reactions. New Rochelle, NY: Medical Letter; 1987.

Schatzberg AF, Cole JO. Manual of clinical psychopharmacology. 2nd ed. Washington, DC: American Psychiatric Press; 1991.

Schou M. Lithium prophylaxis: myths and realities. Am J Psychiatry. 1989;146:573–576.

Slaby AE, Tancredi LR, Lieb J. Clinical psychiatric medicine. Philadelphia: Harper & Row; 1981.

Talbott JA, Hales SC, Yudofsky SC. The American psychiatric press textbook of psychiatry. Washington, DC: American Psychiatric Press; 1988.

VanPragg HM. Psychotropic drugs: a guide for the practitioner. New York: Brunner/Mazel; 1978.

Woods JH, Katz JL, Winger G. Use and abuse of benzodiazepines. JAMA. 1988;260:3476.

Other Resources

Ayd FJ (ed.). International Drug Therapy Newsletter. Ayd Medical Communications, 1130 E. Cold Spring Lane, Baltimore, Maryland, 21239.

Gelenberg AJ (ed.). Biological Therapies in Psychiatry (newsletter). PSG Publishing Company, 545 Great Neck Road, P.O. Box 6, Littleton, MA 01450.

Lithium Information Center University of Wisconsin, Madison, Wisconsin. Tel: (608)263-6171. (Focused literature searches and answers to specific clinical questions.)

Index

Page numbers followed by *f* indicate illustrations.
Page numbers followed by *t* indicate tables.